W9-BOM-943

This book is a gift from the authors.
Please remember to...
"Pay It Forward"
Be well.

More Praise for *The Power of Two*

"As a trial lawyer, Brian Monaghan stood alone—Governor Gray Davis of California once said he would rather wrestle Jesse Ventura than face Brian in trial. In 1998, at the peak of his career, he stood before a massive crowd to receive the Association of Trial Lawyers of America's most coveted award—the Steve J. Sharp Public Service Award; he had just been diagnosed with melanoma. Unbeknownst to the audience, he now faced his last case, the greatest trial of his life, his battle for survival.

The story of how Brian and his wife, Gerri, conquered cancer should be read by anyone with a life-threatening illness. It will make you laugh and cry. . . . It's the greatest tribute to the power of positive thinking since Norman Cousins wrote of his experiences."

—DAVID CASEY, TRIAL LAWYER, FORMER PRESIDENT,
THE ASSOCIATION OF TRIAL LAWYERS OF AMERICA

"By one of America's great trial lawyers, the saga of an extraordinary, successful battle against brain cancer. From a devastating prognosis of months to live, this couple tamed the dragon with courage, intelligence, pluck, humor, and yes, luck. It is a story about the industrial-medical complex of America, with its towering strengths and its frailty.

But mostly it is about the strength of two good people who never stopped believing that they would survive to enjoy their families, friends, and each other. This is a book for all seasons."

—BILL GORHAM, FOUNDER, THE URBAN INSTITUTE, WASHINGTON, D.C.

"With The Power of Two, Brian and Gerri Monaghan have hit one out of the park. This is not only a great story, but it's a winner when it comes to helping all of us cope with cancer or any other tough medical challenge. A tip of my hat to them both!"

—DAVE WINFIELD, BASEBALL HALL OF FAMER

THE POWER of TWO

SURVIVING SERIOUS ILLNESS
with AN ATTITUDE & AN ADVOCATE

by Brian & Gerri Monaghan

WORKMAN PUBLISHING • NEW YORK

A Note to the Reader:
The authors are not, nor do we pretend to be, experts in the medical
field. The knowledge we have acquired and the information shared
with the reader is based on our experience and our common sense. It
is not, and should not be considered, medical advice. We urge you to
consult with and seek treatment from a medical professional. Neither
the authors nor the publisher shall be liable or responsible for any
loss, injury, or damage allegedly arising from any information or
suggestions contained in this book.

Copyright © 2009 by Brian Monaghan and Gerri Monaghan

All rights reserved. No portion of this book may be reproduced—
mechanically, electronically, or by any other means, including
photocopying—without written permission of the publisher. Published
simultaneously in Canada by Thomas Allen & Son Limited.

Library of Congress Cataloging-in-Publication Data is available.

ISBN 978-0-7611-5259-0

Book cover by Janet Vicario
Book interior by Rae-Ann Spitzenberger
Cover photo by Michael Spengler

Workman books are available at special discounts when purchased in bulk
for premiums and sales promotions as well as for fund-raising or educational
use. Special editions or book excerpts can also be created to specification.
For details, contact the Special Sales Director at the address below.

WORKMAN PUBLISHING COMPANY, INC.
225 Varick Street
New York, NY 10014-4381

Printed in the United States of America

First printing March 2009
10 9 8 7 6 5 4 3 2 1

*To each of you who has begun a
journey of your own; you are in our
thoughts and our prayers.*

Acknowledgments

Because our book is a chronicle of our last ten years, space doesn't allow us to give thanks and recognition to all of those who have helped us through this journey. If you are mentioned within these pages, you know that you have played a significant part in our journey. "Thank you" isn't adequate to express what we feel, but we truly do thank you, and again, we thank you.

To our family, most especially our children, Kathi and Tom Vaughn, Patrick and Roseanne Monaghan, Todd and Jennifer Wortmann, and Mark and Sharon Wortmann, and our grandchildren, Dylan and Kyra Vaughn, Jake Monaghan, Trevor and Cassidy Wortmann, and Riley and Reagan Wortmann: there is simply no way we could have gotten through these last ten years without your love and support. You have made the fight worthwhile.

To Gerri's Verge family siblings, Carol, Marion, Bill, Helen, and Diane: although thousands of miles separate us, I always know that you "have my back." To Susan and Steve Parker: you were with us every step of the way, and it goes without saying that you hold a special place in our hearts. Our love and special thanks to "our" cousins, Don and Carol O'Connell, as well as to friends of old, Pat and Jack Durliat, Arch and Carol Woodard, and Clark and Denise Hodgson. A toast to The Lads for always being there, and especially to the first traveling group: Vince Bartolotta, Larry Broderick, Kim Broderick, Dennis Broderick, Terry Broderick, Tim Broderick, Ed Chapin, Brian Forbes, Chuck Fox, Bill Hall, Noel Hall, John Lynch, Mickey McGuire, Dave Monahan, Mike Neil, Terry O'Malley, Mike Reidy, Leo Sullivan, Mike Thorsnes, and Bob Vaage.

And thanks to each of you who at some critical point in our battle stepped in to offer your love and support: Kingsley Aikens, Russ Block, Kim Broderick, Dave and Lisa Casey, Toni and Mark Cincotta, John and Mary Clark, Steve and Rita Conway, Jim Eckman, Emily Einhorn, Lou and Judy Ferrero, Joe and Geri Waranke Kennedy, Jerry and Nancy Kohlberg, Judge Gerry and Laura Lewis, Cathy Lynch, Larry and Stacey Lucchino,

Ceci Doty MacNamara, Jeanie and Jim Milliken, Dan and Mary Mulvihill, Debbie Malloy, Elaine and Rich Murphy, Cathy Philips, Sandra Rockhill, Milt and Maria Silverman, and Sue Young Vaage. A special thanks to Gerri's empathetic listening post, Judith Oakes. Brian's assistants deserve special recognition: Lauren Berry, Shawna Songer, and the best of the best, Vanessa Marshall Praggastis. Brian's thanks for their understanding to the Boards on which he serves: the San Diego Padres, Hastings College of the Law, the American Ireland Fund. We recognize and will always miss two valiant warriors who put up a great fight yet still lost the battle, Judy Keep and Bob MacNamara.

Our thanks to our agent, Linda Chester, whose guidance was instrumental in opening doors for us and for helping us understand the process, and to Karen Olson, who helped give shape to our story and was truly responsible for writing the all-important book proposal. Our thanks to our "book doctor," Kyra Ryan, who helped us to tell our story in our own words, yet was able to help craft those words into a book that will be more easily understood by those who need it most—patients and their advocates. Our thanks to each of the fantastic members of the Workman Publishing team, and especially to Mary Wilkinson, our line editor, Janet Vicario, our book designer, production editor Irene Demchyshyn, and typesetters Barbara Peragine and Jarrod Dyer. And last but not least, to Susan Bolotin, who believed in the value of our story, and not only understood the role of the advocate but became one on our behalf.

Table of Contents

INTRODUCTION

To the world at large, Life is serious but not hopeless.
To the Irish, Life is hopeless but not serious.
—IRISH PROVERB

Brian

I've always considered myself to be one of the luckiest people around, and thought that the phrase "luck of the Irish" was coined to describe my life. But in May of 1998, when I was told I had Stage IV melanoma that had metastasized into two brain tumors and lymph node involvement, I feared that my luck might just have run out.

Stage IV melanoma. There is no Stage V. Doctors told me that without treatment I had three to six months to live. With treatment, maybe a year.

That was ten years ago.

How did I beat these god-awful odds? How did I survive? I'd be lying if I told you that it has been easy. It hasn't. My journey has included a gamma knife procedure, removal of lymph nodes, two craniotomies, being the first recipient of an experimental vaccine, life-threatening blood clots, brain seizures, and aphasia. It has also included the gift of learning to enjoy each and every day.

It's now June 2008. The latest reports from my neurosurgeon and oncologist indicate that my MRIs and CT scans are, once again, "all clear." The last ten years have been an incredible journey, with all of the ups and downs that define a knock-down, drag-out fight to survive.

I've learned a lot along the way. I've learned that qualities that had served me well as a trial lawyer—a never-say-die attitude, a sense of humor—were also invaluable in the fight for my own life. I have an even greater appreciation for the friends, doctors, researchers, lawyers, businessmen, housewives, secretaries, athletes, old people, young children, and even a dog, who all joined the battle at different times and in different ways. Some of the significant individuals who have traveled this journey—doctors, scientists, friends, and family—have graciously added to this book their perceptions regarding the initial diagnosis, the search for a scientific solution, the surgeries, the experimental treatments, as well as their beliefs about why it all worked. I thank them.

Most significantly, I've learned that it's important not to face serious illness alone. Since this journey began, I have come to appreciate more and more with each passing day the importance of having an advocate. When it comes down to it, I was lucky in so many ways and most of all because my wife, Gerri, was with me every step of the way. More than a caregiver, she was my champion, my advocate. She fought for me to get the very best care available, and that made my survival possible. I've had doctors and nurses alike tell me how fortunate I have been to have Gerri in my corner. We've had friends tell us that if they're ever really sick, they want to call on her to be their advocate, too.

In addition to my exceptional advocate and the other people who helped me along the way, I believe my survival is also owed to coincidence, good fortune, and plenty of laughter. I know how damned lucky I am. I also know that my story is not the norm. Not only have I survived and been able to live an absolutely wonderful life, but in my fight against cancer I have been more than blessed with resources not available to many people.

It's an unfortunate reality that too few have the financial capability to seek medical help wherever their research leads them, but I did. Not everyone has the ability to stay at home and rest without the fear of losing his or her job, or, of even greater importance these days, losing medical insurance. I did. Not many people have been able to reap the benefits of access to an emerging vaccine therapy simply because they knew one person who knew another person who knew someone else who was the person developing that very vaccine. But I did. I have certainly been given more than a fair shot in this war against cancer. I've gone into battle with a quiver as well stocked with arrows as anyone has a right to hope for. But one of the ways both Gerri and I filled that quiver was by not hiding from cancer. Instead, we sent out a call for help, and that call was answered. In spades.

In the past few years, we have been contacted by many cancer patients or their advocates, asking us for information or sometimes just hope. Having spent many hours talking with them, I often came away with the sense that there was so much more that I should have said to them about what to do, how to handle it, and reasons for hope.

Gerri and I came to understand more about survival than we ever expected. Once life was back on track for me, I knew I needed a mission. So we decided to write this book to share what we learned. I'm not one to keep my opinions to myself, so in these pages, as I tell what I hope is an inspiring story, you'll also find all my advice for surviving cancer—everything from getting an attitude, or 'tude, to finding a mission that keeps you going when the going gets tough and helps you "pay forward" what I hope will be your good fortune.

Just as important, you'll find Gerri's pointers for advocates. As we got phone calls from people looking for help managing their loved ones' struggles, I listened to Gerri talk with them. Later, I heard her frustration when she knew she hadn't impressed upon these potential advocates the need to speak up for their patients. When we first started writing this book, it was focused on how I survived, and I asked Gerri to explain her role, offering hints about just what she did after my diagnosis and during my several years of treatment. Along the way, we realized that defining the role of the advocate is the most important information we can offer.

We gave an early draft of our manuscript to friends, physicians, and those who had been involved in our battle. We were surprised. Many of them told us that our story was not just about a fight against cancer. Our story offered help and hope for others. Accident victims. Heart attack patients. Anyone involved in a serious medical crisis who needed common sense, a good attitude, and even laughter in dealing with their problem. We learned that our book was less *my* story about fighting cancer, and more *our* story about waging a war against any tough medical challenge.

Unfortunately, the telling of this tale is complicated. It is a story I can write but cannot read. As a result of radiation damage and post-surgical seizures, I now have aphasia, which is the mixing up of words and numbers in rather strange ways. While I can (and do) get outside assistance in reading what I have written, I have again needed Gerri's help. Gerri has helped translate my thoughts and words into more readily comprehensible sentences. Because she was present when critical events occurred, she also understands much of what happened better than I do. She helped me survive—and now she has helped me tell my side of the story. Some early readers of the book have commented that my entries and Gerri's sound quite a bit alike. That may stem from the fact that Gerri has had to act as my "translator," but I think the truth lies somewhere deeper, in that place where couples who love each other live after they've gone through something that changes them forever.

We all know too well the impact that serious illness has had on so many lives. I don't think it's possible to meet a single person who hasn't felt the pain of watching a person they know and love fight an insidious disease or life-threatening condition. As survivors, we want to help by sharing what we learned along the way—our practical ideas and hints, a lot of laughs, a measure of understanding, and something that desperate patients and their loved ones need in fighting their battle: hope.

Our story may not exactly mirror yours, but I know there is much we share. Gerri and I have walked in your shoes. We have been there. We have cried the same tears that you are crying. We have faced the same fears. In writing this book we have one aim: to help you keep strong and keep fighting.

Gerri

Brian has outlived all the dire medical predictions. Talk to any doctor and you will hear the same thing: survival is almost impossible for someone with Stage IV melanoma with two brain tumors as well as tumors in his lymph nodes. Brian went from being a hopeless case to a hope-filled survivor.

Doctors don't like to talk in terms of miracles, and Brian and I are not very religious in the formal sense. With those caveats, Brian's recovery is a miracle. While no one has been able to provide us with a definitive answer as to why Brian is here today, he is here, so we must have done something right.

One thing we do know is that Brian's survival didn't happen without a lot of help—and effort. We know that hearing life-changing words like "cancer" or "car accident" or "stroke" can be devastating and overwhelming, but from the very start, we refused to accept the word "cancer" as a death sentence. From the first days of this battle, we assumed the stance that the best defense is a good offense. We pushed the envelope of medical science as hard as we could, getting second and third opinions, spending a lot of time doing research, and seeking out and then embracing cutting-edge technology and clinical trials.

Early on in our journey, we came up with a shared set of responsibilities. Brian's job was to keep his innate sense of optimism, his joy of life, his belief in his ability to overcome all obstacles, and his hope. My job was to keep him alive. That meant I needed to be more than just supportive and caring. I needed to become his advocate.

While I know that as an advocate I did some things that were really helpful in fighting this battle against cancer, I also don't believe that I did anything extraordinary, anything more than what anyone else in my position would do. I've often told Brian that all I did was use common sense.

"The thing about common sense is that it's not common," was his comeback.

With that in mind, I share my story of being an advocate with others who want to know in their hearts that they are doing all they can to fight for the life of someone they love. Although no one can give us any guarantees on what the outcome will be in fighting cancer or any other serious medical challenge, I can guarantee that any help you provide in your role as an advocate will have an effect on two people: the patient and you. You'll have helped give your loved one an extra edge in fighting this battle. And you'll help yourself by knowing that no matter what the outcome, you were there with him or her, fighting every step of the way. In this book I show how my role as Brian's advocate evolved and offer pointers for advocates, everything from creating a battle plan to making use of university-affiliated medical centers to helping to maintain a patient's dignity.

As we moved through this journey, we became proponents of the idea of "paying it forward." Initially, the idea of writing about our experience held little appeal for me. In fact, Brian had to use all his persuasive powers as a trial attorney to talk me into it. He convinced me by pointing out that perhaps the book could be a way for us to give back some small measure of what we have been given throughout this fight. I came to realize that our struggle wasn't just a battle against cancer, but rather a story of hope against all odds. It wasn't just a fight against a single disease, but the story of a team—a patient and an advocate who fought the battle together.

The reality is that a patient involved in the struggle against cancer or any other major illness is up against the odds. While medical science has come a long way and offers hope for many diseases and illnesses, patients too often find themselves entering life-threatening or life-altering situations in the weakest states they've ever been in. That's where the advocate can step in to speak up for them and give them the extra edge that might make the difference between living or dying.

We advocates come in all shapes and sizes, all ages and all walks of life. An advocate can be a young woman insisting that her baby be given a test her pediatrician is reluctant to order because, despite what she's been told, the mother knows in her heart that something is wrong with her child. An advocate can be a forty-year-old son, logging onto the Internet to find out the best options available for a sick parent who isn't computer savvy. Or he can be an exhausted husband who plants himself next to his wife's hospital bed, hour after hour, day after day, doing everything in his power to ensure that she gets the best medical care possible. An advocate can be a secretary who, watching her friend fighting a disease alone, decides she is willing to step in and become this friend's champion. She can be the desperate wife of a soldier returning from war, fighting the system every step of the way until she finds someone who will listen to her and get her husband the medical care he needs and deserves. By becoming advocates, all these people can make a critical difference in the lives of their loved ones.

Although the disease or situation our loved one is facing may be different, advocates all share the same goal, the goal of doing the best we can for our "patient." We share the need to be there, to constantly ask questions, to not take no for an answer, and above all, to pour our heart and soul into getting the best possible result for those we love. It's with this in mind that I became willing to share Brian's and my story with you.

In this book, we tell the tale of Brian's journey from sickness to health from his point of view and mine. Woven throughout, I share what I learned about being an advocate, including fifty tips to help you help your loved one. It's my hope that in relating our story in this way, you will be both inspired and well-armed with practical advice for what lies ahead.

Brian and I consider laughter to be one of life's blessings, and even in the darkest of times, we always seemed to be able to find our sense of humor. It doesn't hurt that Brian is, in many ways, the quintessential Irishman. A natural storyteller, he loves to laugh and to make other people laugh. This is one of the qualities that first drew me to him, and it's certainly one of the qualities we believe has been a key to his survival.

Here's just one example of how important we think humor can be. Faced with an eight-hour surgery needed to remove a tumor located over the left temporal lobe of Brian's brain, we found a way to laugh. Our very good friends Steve and Susan Parker and I stood surrounding Brian, who looked up at us from his hospital bed in the pre-op ward at the University of California, San Francisco Medical Center. The neurosurgeon and anesthesiologist arrived and again went over the procedure. They assured us that they would do all in their power to make certain that when Brian emerged from the surgery, he would do so with the ability to speak and comprehend. The anesthesiologist asked if we had any questions.

Steve stepped forward and placed his hand on Brian's paunch. "Doctor, can you tell us, When will this swelling go down?"

We all erupted in gales of laughter and as I kissed Brian good-bye, while the shadow of gut-wrenching fear lurked in our thoughts, we both had smiles on our faces.

A few hours later, during our long waiting-room vigil, a man came up to me and told me that he had been in the pre-op area that morning. His wife was there for some fairly routine gallbladder surgery, but she had been crying and very emotional. When they had heard the laughter coming from our cubicle on the other side of a flimsy curtain, she had huffed, commenting, "Those people can't be here for anything important." Now the man standing before me told me that he had just learned the laughter had come from the man with the two brain tumors. He looked me straight in the eye.

"What do you do when things are really serious?" he asked.

I knew the answer to that. This obviously was a very serious time for us, but we were doing the best we could to stick with our goal. We were facing this crisis with laughter and the love of friends.

Today, ten years later, I realize that beyond the love and the laughter, there was another, equally important answer. What did I do when things got very serious for Brian, the man I love? I fought like hell for his life.

Chapter One

GET A 'TUDE

If you can fill the unforgiving minute,
With sixty seconds' worth of distance run—
Yours is the Earth and everything that's in it,
and—which is more—you'll be a Man, my son!

—RUDYARD KIPLING

Brian

D a da dah—*da da* dah—*da da* dah—*da da* dah!
The full-throated sounds of the theme song to *Rocky* reverberated through the building. As soon as I heard it, I charged out of my office and stood at the top of the stairway, arms raised to the sky in full Balboa mode. I don't remember how or when it started, but playing the song that has become the symbol of the underdog fighting against the odds had been adopted by our law firm as our traditional way of facing the first day of trial. Everyone from the receptionist to the attorneys came out of their offices clapping, cheering, and laughing.

To my delight, the look on the face of my client, Dr. Tom Self, transformed from sheer panic at the thought of spending his first day in court to an incredulous, wide-eyed grin. We had achieved the result we were looking for. For a few minutes, at least, fear left his face. We were going up against the odds, but for now, Tom knew his fate was in the hands of a fighter.

Going to trial can be intimidating. No one really likes to go to court—except for that rare beast, the plaintiff's attorney. That

1

would be me. While I thrived in the courtroom, my clients were often at the receiving end of a battle in which everything they had, stood for, or believed in was on the line. Tom Self was no different. It was my mission not to just help him get through this, but as his advocate, to vindicate him and secure a win on his behalf.

I didn't just enjoy what I did for a living. I loved it with a passion. I've always believed that loving what you do is as good as it gets and this is one of the many reasons that, as I've said, I considered myself to be one of the luckiest people I know. But maybe luck isn't really the right word. Raised in an Irish family in a working class neighborhood in Philly, I wasn't exactly born with a silver spoon in my mouth. Looking back, I guess we were lucky that we had spoons at all! From the time I was a kid, I worked hard to get what I wanted. Whether it was summers spent waiting tables, or working my way through law school while supporting a young family, or spending long, long hours preparing a case for trial, I worked damned hard so that I could consider myself lucky. I've always been the eternal optimist. I look at life and see the proverbial glass half full—and somebody is still pouring.

In the spring of 1998, I was at the top of my game. My personal life was wonderful. I was married to a great lady and the fun and excitement generated by our new relationship was only enhanced by the similarity of our backgrounds; it seemed like Gerri and I had been together for years. My kids were doing well and we were all working on integrating two families into one. At fifty-nine, my health was good, and I had great friends to share in some good times. Professionally, I knew I was at the top of my career. I'd been a trial lawyer for twenty-seven years and I was proud of the fact that I had won most of the awards that could be given to a plaintiff's attorney.

As a trial lawyer, you have to be a fighter. It goes with the territory. From early on, I've been able to take some pretty hard knocks, so being a trial lawyer was the perfect profession for me. It's not for nothing that Notre Dame, the "fighting Irish," was my favorite team as a kid. Beyond loving a good fight, I've always enjoyed the sense of fulfillment I got by taking up the cause of people who had been wronged by others. The role of a plaintiff's attorney—my role—was to correct that wrong, and I ate it up.

I played the theme song from *Rocky* for my client's benefit. To get *myself* psyched up for trial, I often watched the opening scene to the movie *Patton*. It's the scene in which the general, played by George C. Scott, stands on stage in front of an enormous American flag and addresses troops about to go to war. He walks in straight and tall, covered in medals. His eyes are clear as he salutes his men.

"I want you to remember," he says after telling the troops to stand at ease, "that no bastard ever won a war by dying for his country. He won it by making the other poor dumb bastard die for his country."

Patton reminds the troops that waging a war requires more than individual effort. "The army is a team," he says. "It lives, eats, sleeps, fights as a team. This individuality stuff is a bunch of crap."

As he scans the room, he acknowledges the fear of going into battle and he tells them he is proud to lead them all into battle anytime, anywhere.

There's something about the scene that never failed to stir me. It grabbed me, helped me focus on the trial ahead, and generated a sense of confidence that I would be able to accomplish what I was setting out to do. It made me stand taller. When I stepped in front of a jury, I always believed completely in the case I was about to present to them. Patton's opening monologue helped me to set the tone, to invoke a sense of inner strength and communicate that to the jury. It was my job to make sure the other poor dumb bastard—the opposing counsel—would "die" for his cause.

Despite the fact that I loved my profession, I knew there weren't too many other trial attorneys who practice into their sixties. And for good reason. The long hours and constant stress take a huge toll. I'd felt this in 1997 after fighting the kind of trial I lived for, a real-life David and Goliath case. The trial itself had been long and grueling—and it had taken a lot out of me. Gerri almost convinced me then that I should retire, and I promised her that I had just tried my last case. But giving up the trial work that I loved was tough for me to accept. I guess I just wasn't ready to "go gentle into that good night."

I have always had a Pavlovian response to a good case with a good client and a great cause. That's why in January of 1998 I broke my promise to Gerri and took on the case of Dr. Thomas Self versus the medical group that employed him. My client had reached a point in his career where he was nationally known as San Diego's father of pediatric gastroenterology. He had been told by the managed group for whom he'd worked diligently for more than fourteen years that he had to "spend less time with his patients" and more time doing expensive, invasive testing on those patients.

But Dr. Self was from the old school. He never forgot that those patients were children, very young children. His years of experience had convinced him that he could often come up with a good diagnosis by utilizing far less invasive and painful tests. But these tests were also far less expensive and—here's the rub—far less lucrative for the managed care entity. Dr. Self refused to conform to the medical group's demands, and for this he was terminated.

His case, highly contested on every level, was defended by three separate law firms. The trial lasted over three months, and in early April 1998 the jury ultimately handed down a $1.75 million verdict in favor of my client. Later, during the second phase for punitive damages, the defendants offered a total of $2.5 million for a settlement to end the case. This case had generated media interest from the beginning and was viewed as a precedent, the first successful outcome for a doctor who had essentially been fired because he had refused to spend less time with his patients. It had significant implications on managed care throughout the country.

As the trial ended, we received numerous requests for interviews. Uncharacteristically, I turned most of these over to my co-counsel, Sherry Bahrambeygui. I was exhausted. We had won an epic battle, but I felt beat, mentally and physically.

Not beaten by opposing counsel, just beat. I don't think I had ever been so tired. After the trial, I caught up on lost sleep and some much-needed exercise but no matter what I did, this all-encompassing weariness didn't go away. A nagging sense of concern began to eat away at the edges of my consciousness.

During the trial's closing argument, I had told a fable about a man losing his reputation through false rumors spread about him. It was a great story that everyone really focused on and enjoyed. In the days that followed the trial, we went to dinner with my daughter Kathi, and Gerri asked me to repeat the story. To my confusion, I couldn't. I drew an absolute blank. I had to turn to Gerri and ask her to tell it. To say that this was unusual is an understatement. I have always seen myself as a storyteller. Now, the stories just wouldn't come.

I was glad that Gerri and I were about to spend two weeks in Puerto Vallarta, Mexico. I was looking forward to her son Mark's wedding, which was to be held there, but I was also telling myself that what I desperately needed—*all* I really needed—was a vacation.

Gerri

"That's a great question. Sherry, why don't you handle that?" said Brian, redirecting a question posed to him by NBC TV correspondent Kelly O'Donnell. In response to another query, he said, "I think it would be great if we let Sherry fill you in on that."

Standing behind the long lines of cable attached to the cameras, I was dumbfounded. What was Brian doing?

It was early April 1998 and my husband was being interviewed for *The Today Show*. A few days before, a jury had come in with a verdict in favor of his client, Tom Self, and this case had generated national media attention from the beginning. Now, after months of grueling effort, seven-day work weeks, and long, long hours, instead of basking in the glow of the Klieg lights, Brian kept deferring to his young co-counsel. I watched, incredulous. By the end of the interview it seemed as if Brian, who, as always, had been lead counsel, was little more than an innocent bystander.

"What's wrong with him?" his secretary, Julie, whispered to me. "This doesn't seem like Brian."

She was right. In the seven years I had known Brian Monaghan, I often teased him about what I called the "microphone principle." Once, I laughingly told him I thought he had been secretly implanted with some kind of a homing device, one that drew him to any mike within a twenty-mile radius. Now with the lights of the national media shining on him, he was uncharacteristically taking a backseat. On our drive home, I questioned him about it. "Brian, what were you doing? You worked so hard on this case. It's been killing you. Why did you keep turning every question over to Sherry?"

His reply calmed me. He reminded me that a year earlier he'd said he would quit the grueling work of a trial attorney and focus his attention on helping the law firm branch out into other fields—and he hadn't kept that promise. The Self trial would truly be his last, he said, and since he was ending his career and Sherry's was just beginning, he wanted to give her all the exposure he could.

Within the next few days, he followed that same pattern, and during interviews with *20/20* and *Good Morning, America,* he constantly turned to Sherry and, in a very gracious manner, asked her to relate the story and the details of the case. I told myself that I was getting what I'd hoped for. His days as a trial lawyer were really over. Now we could move on to a new phase of our life. We had both worked hard, and my plan was for us to start reaping the benefits of that hard work and start playing more.

In all honesty, I had to let go of some residual anger left over from watching Brian push himself too hard yet again during the Self trial. I'd worked as a litigation paralegal, and I knew my sleep pattern was never normal during trials. My mind was on overload, constantly thinking of the case and things we needed to do. Still, I knew I could never fully comprehend just how much stress he or any other gifted trial attorney was under.

Since Brian had reneged on his promise to finish his last trial in 1997, however, I had little sympathy for him. I knew how much he loved the work, but the Self trial had taken a terrible toll, and from my point of view, it was his own darned fault. It was what he had chosen to do. He came home every night absolutely exhausted. If I had served soup, he would have fallen asleep in it. It had always been his practice to begin his trial days at 4:00 a.m., but during this trial he had to drag himself out of bed every morning.

At this point, I really had no concern that Brian's exhaustion was anything other than an expression of his age: he was too old to do trial work. Instead of being afraid, I was angry. I was certain it was the three-and-a-half-month trial that was killing him. When the judge took a five-day vacation, the break was an oasis. As a physician rather than as a client, Dr. Self had watched Brian's condition and thought that perhaps he had some medical problem. He ordered some blood work but the results were negative. We all assumed that Brian had no medical problems other than exhaustion, so I considered our upcoming trip to Puerto Vallarta just what the doctor ordered. My son Mark Wortmann and his fiancée, Sharon Riley, were to be married at our beautiful Ocho Cascadas time-share there, and I was in that happy planning frenzy that mothers go through. Best of all, since I was now convinced that Brian had really tried his last case, I knew that this new phase of our life was about to begin.

Despite all the dire warnings given by *Cosmopolitan* and every other woman's magazine that there weren't any available men for women over forty, in 1995, at the age of fifty-one, I'd married this charming, handsome, fun-loving, intelligent man. Not only did he love me, he embraced (no, he insisted on) accepting my two sons as his own and blending our families into one.

I retired from my work as a paralegal and began to focus on our future. Brian and I lived in a lovely home on the beach in sunny San Diego. We'd been married in this home, in an intimate ceremony surrounded by family and friends. The song we chose for our first dance, "What a Wonderful World" sung by Louis Armstrong, was a clear reflection of the love, hope, and optimism we shared. It all seemed so perfect. I often reminded myself that the life I was living was a long way from the Bronx, where I started out.

Prior to meeting Brian in 1991, I had done some great traveling and really enjoyed it. My grandparents had promised themselves that before they died they would return to the land of their birth, and sadly that had never happened. I had vowed to take that trip for them, so when Brian took me to the Old Sod in the fall of 1993, it was a promise fulfilled. He had been there several times before, so he was the perfect guide. Traveling with a man who has the map of Ireland written all over his face, and who makes friends wherever he goes, was a wonderful experience. I loved listening to the blarney that flew between him and his mates.

Besides the many friends we had, our family was growing, and I was looking forward to grandchildren. I wanted to be the best grandmother ever, and was hoping for the chance to do that while I was still young enough to be an active part of a grandchild's life. Brian's daughter, Kathi Vaughn, and my son Todd Wortmann were both already married to wonderful partners. Although Brian's son Patrick was still single, with my son Mark's upcoming wedding added to the mix, I was optimistic about my chances to be a young grandmother.

It didn't surprise me that during our first ten days in Mexico, Brian spent much of the time quietly reading and catching up on his rest. But he was so quiet that I often asked if he was angry about something. He insisted he wasn't, and was simply taking a backseat so the spotlight could shine on Mark and Sharon and their wedding. And shine it did. The wedding was beautiful.

Still, I felt concerned. Brian is usually the life of any party. In fact, while he waited for me to come down the aisle at our wedding (through no fault of my own I was very late), he kept our guests amused as he regaled the crowd with Irish stories. But this time it was different—at the wedding reception he waved off telling any stories or making any kind of a speech. We were all shocked, especially me.

Once the celebration was over, Brian and I had five days to relax before heading home. It was during these few days in

Mexico that I realized something was really wrong. My antennae came up and haven't gone back down since.

My youngest sister, Diane (I'm the oldest of six), had stayed on after everyone else left, and I asked her to reteach me Setback, a pretty simple card game we'd played as children. Brian had never played it, so she taught him, too. The first time we played, he had trouble grasping the concepts and had her repeat the instructions several times. But he caught on quickly enough that he beat both of us.

The next day, we sat down to play the same game, and it was as if Brian had never played it before. Diane went over the instructions and had to repeat them just as she had done on the previous day. But again he caught on, and again he beat us both.

Before dinner that evening, I pulled Diane aside.

"I'm worried about Brian's memory problems," I said.

She agreed it was strange. "But," she pointed out, "it can't be too bad. He won that game every time."

Although she knew I was worried, I didn't tell her the real source of my concern.

The previous year, 1997, Brian's younger brother Terry had died at age fifty-six. Terry had suffered a type of dementia that affected the frontal lobe of his brain; by the time he died, both his physical and cognitive abilities were those of an infant. His case had been widely studied, and he had been taken to medical centers around the country; the cause was variously attributed to everything from overconsumption of NutraSweet (he had consumed gallons of Diet Pepsi for years) to what we now think is the more likely culprit—head trauma suffered from playing football. Terry had played tackle at Penn State and had been injured early on in his professional career as a defensive end for the Los Angeles Rams.

But back in 1998, all we knew really was that Terry suffered pre-senile dementia. Watching Terry's decline from a successful, good-looking, 6-foot 6-inch, 260-pound hulk of a businessman to a gaunt child had been agonizing for Brian. He often remarked that he would rather die quickly than to live the way Terry had.

Brian also thought that Terry's illness had been an incredible burden on Terry's wife, Mardell, and their four daughters.

As I sat watching a breathtakingly beautiful sunset in Puerto Vallarta, I came to the horrible conclusion that Brian might well be starting down the same road that life had forced on Terry. Was I seeing the beginnings of Brian's slide into dementia? It was an agonizing possibility, but something I had to consider. Because I had no clinical foundation for my belief that something so serious was taking place, I began what has become a pattern for me.

Without causing Brian any undue alarm, I started getting all my ducks in a row. I wanted to find out what was going on with his exhaustion and memory problems before discussing it with him. While never mentioning to him my concerns about the "Terry possibility," as soon as we returned I scheduled Brian for a physical exam with his doctor. I did so under the guise that he had missed his yearly checkup while in trial, and we shouldn't delay in getting it done now.

As always, Brian went off to the checkup by himself and, to my delight, he came home with great news. He had the heart of a lion. His blood pressure and other vital signs were great. His problems with exhaustion could be traced to the rigors of trial. After all, he was feeling much better now, wasn't he? And the memory lapses or problems learning the card games? Well, he was approaching sixty and that stuff happens. He came home with an off-the-cuff diagnosis of "brain farts."

To this day, I believe that Brian likely minimized any problems he was having when he discussed them with his doctor. It is possible he wasn't quite up front about just how much he was forgetting, or as Brian now says, maybe he forgot that he was forgetting.

In any event, this clean bill of health was exactly what I wanted to hear. If a man or woman in a white coat tells you that all is well, you can believe them, right? They are far more intelligent, far better informed, far better educated than you. Or so I kept telling myself, despite a nagging voice in my head that said otherwise.

Now I turned my attention to what I envisioned as the trip of a lifetime. The months spent listening to tapes of Italian lessons were going to pay off. Within a few weeks, we'd be vacationing for a month in Italy with our friends Susan and Steve Parker. A dream come true. And then to top it off, on the way home we were all going to fly to Dublin, where we would meet up with more friends and attend a meeting of the American Ireland Fund, a charity Brian had been working with for many years.

Life was good. No, life was great. Brain farts. I loved it! My relief was short-lived.

Trust Your Intuition

Advocate Tip
#1

For so many people facing illnesses, early diagnosis can make all the difference in the world. Your patient may want to push your concerns onto the shelf labeled "overreacting." I think we all have a tendency to insist that there's nothing wrong, to put off facing the inevitable as long as we can. But when there's a little voice inside you insisting that something is amiss, you need to listen to it. Isn't it better to be labeled an overreactor than to spend the rest of your days mourning the fact that if you had trusted your instincts, you might have been able to help achieve a better outcome? So listen to your personal Jiminy Cricket— he just might help you save a life.

Brian

On Wednesday, May 20th, 1998, just a little more than a week after that first visit to the doctor, I woke up with a weird feeling. For the preceding several days, I'd had a series of migraine headaches. Bad ones. Since I had experienced headaches for years, initially they weren't a cause for concern. But today was different. It was as if I was in a fog, one that just wouldn't clear. I couldn't mentally put together what was going on, and try as I might I couldn't hide my confusion.

Gerri sat down next to me on the bed. "Brian, can you add 50 and 27?" she asked.

I couldn't, so just like the kid in school who keeps stalling while hoping to remember the answer, I responded, "Why are you asking?"

That didn't fly with Gerri. I kept asking her to repeat the question while I kept hoping I'd be able to come up with the answer. I couldn't.

Alarmed, Gerri immediately called our friend Dan Einhorn, a physician, and told him what was going on. Within an hour, Dan had arranged for me to be seen by a neurologist he considered to be the best around.

By the time I met with Dr. Joel Kunin that afternoon, my comprehension abilities were back to normal. I had no problems with words or numbers, and I was sure Gerri had overreacted. Since my speech and cognitive abilities were all normal, Dr. Kunin initially felt I probably had a transient ischemic attack (a very mild stroke), but I seemed to have recovered from it with no problem. As an extra precaution, he ordered an MRI of the brain for the following morning.

The rest of that day was uneventful, and since I was once again doing well, I felt pretty good about the preliminary diagnosis of a mild stroke. The good feeling I had didn't last long.

I had the MRI the next morning. Stuffing my 6-foot 3-inch, 220-pound frame into that small cylinder wasn't easy, but luckily I don't have any of the problems with claustrophobia that affect many people. Although the words "MRI of the brain" should have bothered me, I don't remember being overly concerned. Somehow I was able to shove any fear to the back of my mind.

After the MRI, I drove back to the office and immediately began an important meeting scheduled to last all day. My law partners and I were looking into taking our firm in a completely new direction involving complicated insurance fraud and corporate malfeasance cases. This was something I had been working on for months, even while I was in trial. It was really important to me—I saw it as a way to keep the law firm viable as I stepped down from trial work.

In the early afternoon I was called out of the meeting and told I had a phone call from Dr. Einhorn.

"Brian, I've got the results of your MRI test and I need to go over them with you. I want you to come to my office immediately," he said, his usually relaxed voice taking on a certain urgency. There was a pause before he added, "And you are not to drive."

Dan said he'd left a message for Gerri and he believed that she was already on her way to pick me up.

Dan's admonition not to drive gave me a sinking feeling in the pit of my stomach. I went back to the meeting and asked Sherry Bahrambeygui, the partner who had been so helpful in the Self trial, to step outside with me. I told Sherry that my MRI had apparently caused some concern and that I was leaving immediately to see Dr. Einhorn.

"Don't alarm the others," I said. "I'll fill them in when I get back. I'll see you later this afternoon."

Looking back, I realize how unrealistic, how totally unprepared I was for what was to follow.

In the car I asked Gerri for any more information that Dan might have given her, but she didn't know anything. We were scheduled to leave for our month-long trip to Italy in two days, and she'd been having her hair done when she got Dan's message on her cell phone. The words he'd had for her—"Don't let Brian drive"—were enough to keep us both in strained silence.

When we checked in with Dr. Einhorn's receptionist, I noticed she didn't engage in our normal back-and-forth banter, but instead gave me a quiet smile. Although there were other patients waiting ahead of us, she immediately took us into Dan's office, saying, "The doctor is waiting for you."

Dan came around from behind his desk and greeted us more formally than usual, his perennial warm, wide smile nowhere to be seen.

He perched on the edge of his desk. We sat down in two chairs across from him.

"Brian, we know the reason for the headaches and the problems with memory and words that you have been having," Dan Einhorn said. "The MRI shows two brain tumors."

Total silence. No shrieks. No cries.

My training as a trial lawyer has given me the ability to take body blows without a trace of emotion, and I guess that training kicked in because I don't recall showing any outward reaction. I think I remember Gerri reaching for my hand, but other than that, I was totally stunned. I had known something was wrong, but brain tumors? *Two* brain tumors?

He asked me whether I had any history of cancer.

"No," I replied.

Gerri almost jumped out of the chair. "Brian, yes you did. Don't you remember? You had that melanoma spot on your back three years ago!"

"But they cut that out and it was all taken care of," I replied.

Back in 1995, I had gone to my doctor about a spot in the middle of my back. He'd sent me to a surgeon who cut out a huge area for what looked like a small dark pencil point. The pathology report said it was melanoma, but it also said that the margins of the huge incision were all clear of any cancer. To me, "all clear" meant all clear. I had dealt with it and it was over. Done. That's how I always handled problems. Take care of them and move on.

In many respects, this was the same approach I took to life in general. When dealing with anything medical, it allowed me to keep doing my job and keep living my life without worry. But by dismissing my recent history with cancer, I wasn't helping the doctor figure out what was wrong with me. It was Gerri who was helping.

Write Down the Medical History

Advocate Tip **#2**

It's so important that you know your patient's medical history in detail, and what's more, that you have a written record of it. Everyone should take the time to write down his or her own history, as well as that of family members, as soon as possible, even before illness strikes. We all forget things when we get to the doctor's office—What medicines are you taking? In what dosage? Does heart disease run in your family?—and having a written record to refer to can mean you are able to provide the kind of details that help doctors do their jobs better. See page 195 for an example of the information that should be included in a basic medical history.

Much of our meeting with Dan Einhorn was a blur for me, but Gerri later told me that when she mentioned the word "melanoma," a look of deep concern had flashed across Dan's face.

We walked quietly to the car, and Gerri assumed her new position in the driver's seat. I had a sense of complete disconnect. While I kept repeating the words "brain tumors" over and over to myself, I had a hard time letting them actually sink in. For a few minutes we just sat there and held on to each other in stunned silence. It was as if, from outside the car, tremendous pressure was bearing down all around us. But inside, sitting next to my wife, I felt safe. I knew I hadn't married just a pretty face; I had known from the first time I met Gerri that she had incredible inner strength and could be a force to be reckoned with. Now, she pulled away from me and quickly blinked back tears from those blue eyes I loved. Her strength took over, and what she said to me in that dark moment resonates with me to this day.

"Bear," she said, "however long we have, whatever time we have, we are going to deal with this with two things: laughter and love. I'm willing to bet that in whatever time we have left, people we know will die in car accidents or keel over from heart attacks. We are going to have the ability to cherish and really appreciate each and every day. We are going to love and laugh and fight this. And you are going to win."

To this day, those words of hers remain the most powerful of any I have ever heard.

Over the years, I've learned that each of us deals with a crisis in our own way. My way was to get a 'tude. The phrase is one that I picked up somewhere in sports, and it goes far beyond the simple idea of an attitude. It's about reaching deep down inside to find courage, toughness, resilience, humor, and passion.

From Lance Armstrong, who overcame Stage III testicular cancer and went on to win the Tour de France seven times, to the guy down the street who has overcome incredible odds in beating cancer, I have found that a winning attitude is a common trait among survivors. Doctors, nurses, therapists—all of them will tell you that an invincible spirit can't always overcome the odds. But, boy, it sure can help.

There are some people who truly believe they can beat this disease, and I'm one of them. When doctors, a few weeks after my initial diagnosis, would tell me I had a 15 percent chance of survival, I have to tell you in all honesty, I really felt bad for the other 85 percent of the patients who weren't going to make it. Gerri has told me many times that if we could bottle that attitude and give it to others, it would be the greatest gift we could pass on. Along with many of our doctors, she and I will always be convinced that my attitude helped tremendously.

But then, I've always been a fighter.

Maybe it started with Tony, a bully in my neighborhood who was older and bigger than I was. It was during World War II, and while my father was away in the navy we lived in an apartment in a blue-collar neighborhood in Philly. One of my first clear memories is of being on the blacktop basketball court across from our apartment when Tony suddenly punched me. My guess is I was probably about five or six.

I vividly remember coming home crying, my nose running. My mother met me at the front door. She knelt down on the floor beside me.

"Tony beat me up!" I cried.

"Did you hit him back?" my mom immediately asked.

I continued whining, "He beat me up."

When I acknowledged that I hadn't hit him back, my mother reacted in a way that wouldn't win today's Good Housekeeping Seal of Approval, but it was certainly how people dealt with problems in a working class neighborhood during World War II. She told me to go back to Tony, to walk straight up to him and punch him in the nose.

I whined even louder, "But he's going to beat me up again."

She was adamant. So I went back to Tony and his friends and followed her instructions. I don't think I even landed a punch before Tony walloped me again. My mother had watched the "fight" from afar, and this time when I came home she hugged me and gave me all the love a little kid needs. She told me that she was proud of me, but then came the tough part. I was ordered to go up to Tony every time I saw him and, without giving him any warning, hit him in the nose. That order brought a great deal of pleading—I didn't want to get beat up again. But when my mother said something, it was going to be done. She even found someone to teach me how to land a punch.

From then on, whenever I saw Tony, I would walk up and take a shot at him. I don't remember ever winning any of those fights, but I do remember that eventually he began to avoid me whenever he saw me. Since he was known as the toughest kid in the neighborhood, I didn't have any problems with any of the other kids.

Years later, when I played football at LaSalle High, I was in on all the fights. Clark Hodgson, a teammate and a good friend to this day, says that whenever the whistle blew away from the ball, he came to know without looking that Monaghan was in another fight. That tenacity may have resulted in my being recruited to play football at the United States Naval Academy.

Now I was going to take the same tough approach in fighting for my life.

"*We're* going to win," Gerri went on to say, turning to me in the car. I had a sense of great strength from her. Rocky Balboa and General Patton, meet Gerri Monaghan! She gave me a little smile, a light kiss, and another long hug. Then she started the car and we were on our way. At that moment, we began a journey that has lasted more than ten years.

Gerri

The moment Dan Einhorn said "brain tumors," Brian and I both reacted with outward calm. But inside, those words hit me with the force of a tsunami. I felt as if I'd been kicked in the stomach. I had to keep swallowing to fight the nausea.

For a moment I chose to remain still, like a child hiding under the covers, secure in the belief that if you can't see people, they can't see you. But while I could freeze myself emotionally for a few moments, I couldn't stop the inevitable. Our lives had changed forever.

A good friend and a brilliant physician, Dan is a specialist in endocrinology, not oncology. It was because he is an incredibly kind, caring individual, and because of our friendship, that he had taken it upon himself to give us the terrible diagnosis. "Brain tumors," he said. But he also gave us the first word of the beginning of our new life. As we left his office, he gave me a hug, and whispered one simple word into my ear: "Courage."

"Courage" became a mantra for me over the next few days, weeks, and months. It was a word I repeated to myself many times while waiting for MRI results, CT scan (also known as CAT scan) reports, and during the long hours spent in surgical waiting rooms.

When I recall that first moment now, more than ten years later, a shiver still runs through me. There is never a reason to tell someone to have "courage" unless you know that person really needs it. I did.

Advocate Tip
#3

Gather Your Courage

There is no one better at taking up causes than my husband. It was no coincidence that the 4-foot glass etching in the lobby of his office was of St. George, whose long sword is piercing a dragon under the feet of his horse. St. George is representative of who Brian was as a lawyer, and still is as a man: he is a bold Dragon Slayer. As a plaintiff's lawyer (and damn proud of it), he was always on the attack, with his cause figuratively emblazoned on his shield.

Brian entered the courtroom with a passion for his clients and a belief in their cause. Throughout his years of legal advocacy, he was able to convince jury after jury of the merits of his case, not just with attention to detail, hard work, or great oratorical skills, but also with deep passion. He was, without fail, "goal-line oriented." His faith in his mission allowed him to visualize the goal of winning, and he allowed nothing to get in the way. But for now, my St. George wasn't able to pick up his sword, let alone swing it.

I would have to pick up that sword myself.

"Courage," Dr. Einhorn said. I've never thought of myself as courageous, perhaps because I thought of courage in the physical sense. On any normal day, there isn't enough money in the world to convince me to parachute out of an airplane, or leap off a platform with my ankles attached to a bungee cord. I'd rather spend the winter on a mountaintop waiting for the spring thaw than to ski down a double black diamond slope.

So perhaps courage is nothing more than doing something outside the ordinary, something beyond what you usually do. I think that you do whatever you need to do to help the person you love. You find courage, and you come up with a plan. When there's a crisis at hand, there's a need to get something done. Curling up in the fetal position isn't an option, if you want to fight for the life of the person you love.

As we left the doctor's office, I understood why the nurses had turned their eyes away from us when we arrived. They had known. The fact that they couldn't face us made the enormity of the diagnosis even greater. As we left, Dan showed us a side door so we could leave without having to face anyone else. Brian and I stood in an empty corridor and held each other. For a long time, neither of us spoke.

I'm a down-to-earth person, and the need to deal with reality quickly took hold. The nurses in Dr. Einhorn's office didn't have to face the reality of Brian's cancer, but I did. Although this battle against cancer began when we had been married only a few years, we had such similar backgrounds that we really had the same approach to dealing with the problems each of us faces in the normal course of our lives. I had seen Brian succeed over and over again in trial. Now it was my time to step up and join him. His trial had become my trial.*

* For Dr. Dan Einhorn's perspective on how Gerri handled the diagnosis, see page 205.

In the car I told Brian we would face it all with laughter and love, and that we were going to fight this cancer and win.

As I recall these words now, I sometimes wonder where they came from. I know how devastated and frightened I was, and I ask myself, How did I do that? How could I be so strong?

It's because there simply were no acceptable alternatives. There were only two possibilities: fight or flight. I chose to fight.

Chapter Two

GET AN ADVOCATE

If you think you're too small to have an impact,
try going to sleep with a mosquito.
—ANITA RODDICK

Brian

After leaving Dan Einhorn's office, as we drove in silence most of the way home, I tried to focus on Gerri's words of encouragement. They were deeply comforting. But Gerri's strong words aside, it is obvious to me now that I wasn't ready to deal with the enormity of my situation. I had spent fifty-nine years on this earth as a hard-driving, type-A personality, and that didn't change with the simple words "brain tumors." By the time we were nearing home, I was absolutely certain that what needed my immediate attention was . . . my law practice.

I told Gerri—who had worked with me at the office until we started seeing each other—that instead of going home I wanted to join the others in the meeting. She thought I was crazy. I had to convince her that we just couldn't leave those people there waiting for me. Even at this critical moment, as had happened all too often in the past, my legal practice came first. I didn't realize it yet, but if I was to survive, I was going to have to learn to change that focus. And change it fast.

Reluctantly, Gerri went with me to the meeting, which had moved from the office to a restaurant overlooking San Diego

Bay. We were the last to arrive and joined the other four lawyers already sitting at an umbrella table. By now it was about four o'clock so we had the place almost to ourselves. It was the kind of day that had drawn me to San Diego more than thirty years ago, with perfect weather, clear blue skies, and sailboats gliding back and forth in front of us.

Never one to mince words, I cut right to the chase. "The MRI shows that I have two brain tumors," I told them straight out. "They don't know much more than that right now, but there's some concern that it might be melanoma."

Deafening silence.

Immediately, Sherry Bahrambeygui got up and ran from the table. With a strong background in medicine, she was the first to realize the impact of my words.

The others began peppering me with questions, mostly along the lines of, "What are they going to do for you?"

I had no answers for them. None at all. Dan had told us that he would make some calls to other doctors and would call us back first thing in the morning. For now, we didn't know much.

Watching the looks on the faces of my colleagues and seeing tears in their eyes helped me realize the terror I was facing. One by one, they took turns leaving the table—later I learned that they were going off to "collect" themselves. One by one, they insisted that our plans for the law firm were inconsequential.

I fell back into my role of senior partner. As the guy who had always been the head of the firm, I tried to reassure them that things would go on as usual. I said we would have to put our plans for major expansion on hold right now, but we could get back to it just as soon as I had taken care of the brain tumors. Everyone seemed to have a better handle on the reality of my situation than I did. They each told me that getting well should become my focus, and they offered to help in any way they could. Then each of them spent time giving Gerri hugs and words of encouragement. Pretty soon, the meeting was over. It was time for me to begin to deal with my new reality. My life had changed and there would be no going back.*

*To understand more about how Brian "wrote the ending first," see Sherry Bahrambeygui's comments on page 204.

21

People always ask me, "How did you deal with cancer? When you found out that you had brain tumors and only had a couple of months to live, what did you think? How did you react? What did you do?"

Early on, I'm not sure that I could have said exactly how I was dealing. I wasn't feeling well enough to deal with much more than being sick and responding to gut reactions and needs. Since then, I've read a lot and can tell you that I did not exactly experience the stages that Elisabeth Kübler-Ross described in her watershed book *On Death and Dying*. But a discussion of those stages is a good way to explain more about the approach I adopted.

According to Dr. Kübler-Ross, the five stages are:

1) Denial—refusal to accept what has happened;
2) Anger—"How could this have happened to me?" Or simply, "Why me?";
3) Bargaining with God—"I'll be good if only you save my life";
4) Depression—needs no further explanation; and
5) Acceptance—"It's time to get ready and do what needs to be done."

I speak purely from personal experience here, but I think the process of dealing with those five stages can take too much time and energy. There is much to be done in your effort to survive or, in the worst case, enjoy the time you have left. Spending too much time worrying about the stages of your illness takes away from the ability to focus on recovery. If you're in a fight for your life, I recommend skipping straight to acceptance. Again, maybe it was my hard Irish upbringing that gave me this tough attitude but, to be honest, my response to each of those five stages goes something like this:

1) Denial. Within an hour of my diagnosis, I was absolutely certain that what needed my immediate attention was my law practice. I don't understand the psychology of how it works, but I think that our minds are such that we can only begin to accept the reality of a situation in small doses. It's probably what keeps us from falling down and screaming, "No, this can't be true." At least that's how it worked for me. It's obvious that my immediate

reaction of having to get back to the office was denial on some level. But complete denial is a luxury that can't last long. You have been given a grim diagnosis. This is real. You can allow yourself some downtime, some time to accept the reality of your situation. But you don't have long. Soon you'll have to splash the cold water of reality on your face. It's time to move forward.

2) Anger. Have you ever had your pocket picked or your car scratched? Have you gotten angry about a political decision while recognizing that you have no ability to affect the outcome? On those occasions did you feel angry, then frustrated, then angrier? Get a life! Move on! Don't waste your valuable energy. There's just too much to do—if you really want to survive.

3) Bargaining with God. You'd probably have a better impression of me as a person if I could tell you that my initial thoughts on getting diagnosed were to reach out to my Creator and ask for help. But I wouldn't be telling the truth. Though I was raised as a devout Catholic, by the time my cancer came along I had stopped any formal praying. I firmly believe that if you don't pray to God on good days, you shouldn't pray when things aren't going well. Later, when friends and family would offer prayers, I happily accepted their love and attention. But how could I bargain with God? I'd be a hypocrite if I now asked God to allow me to live. I was willing to rest my case on the evidence. I had lived a pretty good life in trying to follow the Golden Rule. What God did with me now was up to Him. I didn't feel I had much bargaining power in our relationship!

4) Depression. I was very fortunate. There were times I got the blues after my diagnosis, but they didn't last long. Whenever I found myself feeling down, I asked myself, Am I a wimp? Do I really want to live? Or would I rather waste what time I have left mooning about a terrible situation? I made a conscious effort to think about how lucky I was in comparison to some young child who might die without having been blessed with the years and the many gifts I had been given.

I realize, however, that depression can be serious, and if that's the case for you, by all means get help quickly. But *carpe diem*— seize the day—is an attitude I love, and with the realization that our days are limited, with or without cancer or any other medical bogeyman lurking in the background, it's an attitude I think is worth adopting.

5) Acceptance. My attitude has always been, This is the way it is. When an important witness during a trial suddenly becomes unavailable (or any number of other obstacles occur in the course of a trial), what does a trial lawyer do? Does denial, anger, or depression inhibit the attitude of "get on with it" or "let's find an alternative"? No. My attitude has always been, What do I have to do now to make this work? For me, it all boils down to the simple idea that if you want to live, there are lots of decisions to make; there are many things that you need to accomplish. Especially early on, I found it was better to act than to feel. Accept that you are facing an extremely difficult situation, and deal with it!

The most important thing I could do to deal with my cancer now was to accept Gerri's help.

By the time Gerri and I left Dr. Einhorn's office, it had become obvious to me that I would not be able to competently advocate for myself, despite the fact that I had been an advocate for others throughout my life. When I sat with my colleagues in that restaurant, too, I could feel my own role as chief counsel slipping away. I was becoming more like one of my clients now.

Here's how it worked. When potential clients came into my office for the first time, they needed desperately for someone to take control of a situation that they had not confronted in their lives. No matter what the legal problem—a wrongful termination, a personal injury action, an antitrust action—they usually had a sense of confusion, desperation, and often anger. Always, they were under enormous pressure. And as long as my client was direct and honest with me, I'd assume most of the pressure. As an advocate, I insisted that my client relax and let me do the job. I spent my career training clients to accept this kind of help.

Suddenly, with the diagnosis of Stage IV melanoma with metastasized tumors, I desperately needed an advocate myself, someone who could be in control and take responsibility for the case of a very strong-minded person. Gerri was the person I trusted for the job.

Gerri and I had met in 1991 when she applied for a position as a paralegal at my law firm in San Diego. Since it was close to lunchtime, I asked her to join me for a get-acquainted meal. We walked to a nearby sports-theme restaurant and it quickly became apparent that she had a vast knowledge of sports. I considered myself to be a huge fan, but she blew me away with her storehouse of sports trivia. During lunch, we talked baseball and football. Gerri told me of her belief that when you spend your early years in New York City, as she had, you either love sports or despise them. She loved them. In fact, she told me that while growing up, she thought the New York Yankees were the host team for the World Series every year and the other team was just invited to play them.

We discovered that we had even more in common. Both of us had been raised on the East Coast in Irish families, Gerri in New York City and Manchester, Connecticut, and I in Philadelphia. We liked the same books and music, and both of us loved the legal profession and loved to laugh. We shared a bond of being single parents. I had raised Kathi and Patrick in San Diego since my divorce in 1978. Gerri's sons, Todd and Mark, had been raised in Colorado, but after her divorce and with both of them in college, she had moved to San Diego. All four of our children were within three years of each other in age.

I hired her and within a short time recognized that she was the best paralegal I had ever seen in my twenty-seven years of practice. Not only was she great at her job, she was a fun, quick-witted person. In no time, Gerri became my best friend. I even went to her for advice on my various romances.

I'm not a complete idiot, and I had certainly noticed that among her other attributes, Gerri is a very pretty woman with the most beautiful blue eyes. But I wasn't interested. Not me. I had a long-standing rule that you don't mix business with pleasure, and I wasn't about to change. Hell, as an employment law specialist, I had preached that same rule to my clients for years. So while our friendship continued to grow, I continued to view it as simply that—friendship. I didn't even realize I was in denial.

One day, Gerri suggested we get together for dinner. We sometimes did that, usually spending the time discussing a case we were working on, or our children. This time, however, as we finished a pleasant dinner, Gerri said, "Brian, I'm giving you my notice. I'm quitting. I've decided that I can't work for you anymore."

I was shocked.

"Ger, what are you thinking? You have a great job. Our cases are the most interesting anywhere. I must be the best boss in the world. If it's money, you know I'll take care of that. What could be the problem? How could you want to quit?"

"I've become involved with someone," she said.

"Who?" I asked. I was astounded. Outraged. Confused.

"You!"

I swear that on a conscious level, I had never thought about that possibility. She was my friend. Damn it, she was my employee! But I couldn't stand the thought of not having her in my life. We spent the next hour or so talking about how much we enjoyed our time together. The more we talked, the more I realized that the woman I wanted to spend my life with was sitting right in front of me. My years of being a serial monogamist were receding before my eyes.

We both knew that dating each other would be awkward, and so before it became "public," I went from office to office and sat down with everyone in the firm, from receptionist to partner, and told them Gerri and I were going to start dating. The answer was, typically, "Dummy, what took you so long!"

The feelings I had so long ignored came to the surface. Within no time it was easy to acknowledge the love we shared, and in September of 1995 we were married.

At a birthday dinner for Gerri several years earlier, I had asked her sons to tell me a story about a moment that made them proud of their mother. They said there were many to choose from, but together they agreed on one. Sometime in the mid-1980s Todd and Mark were driving into the city of Grand Junction, Colorado, from their home about five miles out of town. They were caught in traffic because of an accident, got out of the car, and walked up to the top of a hill to see what they could do to help.

Just then, a police car pulled up and the officer asked, "What's going on down there?"

A man who had been watching the entire scene said, "A kid on his bicycle has been hit by a car down at the bottom of the hill; an ambulance has already been called."

"Who's in charge?"

"The lady in the yellow tennis dress. She's taking care of the boy and seems to have everything in control."

"I'll go have traffic rerouted in both directions."

"She's already sent people to do that."

Mark and Todd looked at each other, walked a little farther, and surveyed the scene. They had both suspected immediately that the lady in the yellow tennis dress who had taken charge and had everything under control was their mother. It was.

Who could possibly be a better advocate for me? I knew my wife could and would do it right. Gerri was bright and strong. She was motivated and, what's more, she happened to love me.

Understand That Advocates Come in Many Forms

Advocate Tip
#4

One of Brian's doctors, Joe Fay, once told me, "No one has more of a vested interest in helping a loved one than you do." And in Brian's case, the best advocate he could have did turn out to be me; other patients, however, find great advocates in their adult children, siblings, parents, friends, and even professionals.

While I believe the best advocate for a patient is the person he or she is closest to—probably you, if you've picked up this book—there is obviously a strong need for advocates in whatever form. Indeed, several for-profit companies have recently sprung up to meet that need. But professional advocacy is a brand-new concept; as of yet, no one regulates these companies, and virtually anyone can promote himself as an advocate. So although you may not be a "professional," I think that your level of interest, care, and concern can more than make up for your lack of medical knowledge.

Still, if you feel that you and your patient need more support, try contacting the social worker in your local hospital, or the American Cancer Society, American Heart Association, or whatever health-related entity would apply to your patient's situation. These groups often have information about patient advocacy organizations that can provide assistance.

Gerri

As we left the restaurant, the hugs and words of encouragement from our friends and colleagues helped, but nothing could cushion us from the hard, cold reality of the diagnosis.

That night, Brian and I made the essential calls we needed to make. We called our children and a few friends and relatives. The common reaction was stunned silence. Most weren't quite sure what melanoma meant, but the words "brain tumors" have the same effect on everyone—the feeling of being punched in the stomach, of the air being sucked from your lungs.

Advocate Tip #5

Don't Let Others' Reactions Get You Down

Although all the people I talked to that night were very supportive, this would not always be the case further along in our journey. In talking to other advocates, I've learned that one of the things we all share is our incredulity at the reactions we've received from "outsiders." Prepare yourself. It's a fact of life that people often say the most tasteless things, often not meaning to, but usually getting the same reaction from the recipient: shock, disbelief, with anger close behind.

"Don't give him false hope. You can't afford to be this optimistic right now. False hope is the worst thing either one of you can have."

"You must feel so guilty about not being there when he had the seizure."

And my favorite: "He's not going to get out of this alive!"

My reply to that one was, "You know what, neither are you. None of us will." After all, none of us is destined for immortality.

It's likely that you'll hear some similar statements. As an advocate, try to understand that these individuals are really not proposing that you act without optimism, act as if it's hopeless, or believe that you are responsible for everything that goes wrong. But while they may not be acting with malice, it's very easy for their comments to get under your skin. I know that they did with me. I've had to talk myself into realizing that it's the same thing people experience when they lose a loved one. Well-meaning people say things like "It's really for the best," and they truly don't mean to offend. Sometimes they are just clueless.

But although I'm willing to give these people the benefit of the doubt, I don't think I need to give them the time of day. Walk away if that's your style, or speak out if that serves you better. If you have the nerve and the style to carry it off without being offensive, you might say, "I really don't think that you can understand our situation at all. But I know that you're not trying to be hurtful so I'll thank you for the good thoughts you have for us." I wish I had the sense to have said things like that.

One thing you should *not* do is share these thoughtless comments with your patient. I knew that Brian had enough battles to wage without getting involved in this one, and there simply wasn't anything to gain by passing the comments along to him. It is, however, a good idea to get it off your chest by telling someone you trust. Just remember that you're doing the best that you can, and the "outsiders" truly have no idea of what you and your patient need to do to get through each day.

Later, after I got Brian to bed, I walked outside and looked back into the house. It was very quiet and almost completely dark. I felt as if I was in some kind of mourning and yet I knew that I couldn't give in to that feeling. I needed to shake it off. I was exhausted but couldn't go to sleep. I had to do something.

I knew that the first part of this fight would depend largely on me. Brian is a fighter by instinct, and I was sure that he wouldn't give up without a tremendous battle. I could do no less for him. We were going to war prepared to do everything in our power to win. That first night I realized, just as Brian had, that we needed to get a 'tude. From the very beginning, that attitude would keep us on the offense, not defense. It was a great thought but neither of us had any kind of a medical background and really no idea what that offense should be. Even so, I knew one simple thing: every battle needs a plan, and this battle was no different. I went back inside, got a yellow legal pad, sat down at the kitchen table, and wrote out a plan of attack.

Create a Battle Plan

Your battle plan will vary depending on the situation your loved one is in, but I found that the basics apply across the board, and the very act of forming a plan is helpful. I wrote down several categories, or battle fronts:

• **Research:** Initially, my thought process was pretty basic—you've got to know your enemy. So the first thing I wrote was, "What is melanoma?" It was vitally important for me from day one to learn as much as I could about the cancer we were facing.

• **Physicians:** There are lots of doctors in the world, but they're not all equal. I wanted the best doctors I could find for Brian, and I needed help in finding out who was the best. I called Ginny Nelson, a longtime friend and an exceptional medical malpractice attorney. I thought that Ginny could provide some helpful insights, and she did. You'll likely get recommendations from many people, all with the best of intentions, all telling you that the person they are recommending is absolutely the best. It's not going to be easy to go against a recommendation from someone you know, but after checking a doctor out from as many different sources as you can, you have to use your gut instinct to find the doctor who is right for you. If all else is equal, it's always nice to choose the doctor with the best bedside manner. You will be going through hell, and it helps to actually like the person you're dealing with. Even so, I'd rather work with someone capable of putting out fires, than with someone who says soothing things as we go down in flames.

• **Nutrition:** We already ate right in a general attempt to stay healthy and avoid illness, so it seemed logical to me that we could look at diet as a way to help Brian fight cancer. My thought was that there had to be something we could do to help his immune system. I decided we would pursue every avenue of help we could imagine, and I knew I needed to learn about vitamins, dietary supplements, and disease-fighting nutrients beyond vitamin C.

• **Communication Network:** Brian had a large and far-flung "band of brothers" in addition to our relatives and close friends, and I knew that we would want to be in communication with everybody who might want to help. I also knew that trying to keep in touch with all these people could consume me. So, going back to my days as a room mother from my sons' elementary school classes, I set up a telephone tree. I arranged to have one person in charge of each branch, and that person became our conduit to the rest of their group. It sounds simple, but it is really vital. Your "Brian" is going to need all the sleep he can get, and much as people want to help, you'll both be worn out in no time if you call everyone who wants to hear how he's doing. Now that we've become computer savvy, we've found that e-mail lists of people provide a great way of communicating with everyone. It's fast, effective, keeps everyone in the loop—and you won't lose your sanity in the process.

After I wrote down these four personal battle fronts, I noted beside each one the names of people—friends, acquaintances, friends of friends, family—I thought could be of help in that area. Among the few things I knew for certain that first evening was that just as Brian couldn't do it all himself, I couldn't do this by myself either. No one can. Not even you. For help with your own battle plan, see page 201.

Recently, I found the manila folder I started that night and laughed when I read the label: To the War. "To the war" was a phrase used by Brian's partner Mike Conger, and it was often heard when the firm was gathering its forces to deal with what Brian always described as the "dark side." It became my personal slogan, and it should become yours as well.

All these years later, I must admit that what I did that night surprises me. It seems so strong on my part. Looking back, I realize it probably wasn't strength as much as my need to simply do *something*. While Brian slept, I started doing things by instinct. I didn't know that what I was doing had a name, but that night I began my new life as an advocate. I couldn't guess who or what would come into our lives during our war against Brian's cancer, but by the time I crawled into bed, quietly wrapped myself around him, and fell into an exhausted sleep, I knew I had done what I could to start us marching.

Chapter Three

ISSUE A CALL
TO GENERAL
QUARTERS

A journey of a thousand miles begins with a single step.

—CONFUCIUS

Brian

In the days and weeks following my diagnosis, Gerri and I called on all the resources we had. My style of dealing with problems has been shaped in part by my military experience, and that old training came in handy now. After I graduated from the Naval Academy in 1962, I spent five years serving on board destroyers, often patrolling off the coast of North Vietnam. One of the first things you learn on board a ship is the concept of a call to general quarters. This alarm would sound throughout the ship, calling all hands on deck to respond to an emergency, whether it be a torpedo boat maneuvering to fire on us or a pilot shot down in the water.

When I got the diagnosis of Stage IV melanoma, Gerri and I, in effect, issued a call to general quarters. Because we sounded a general alarm, word of my diagnosis was spread far beyond our family and close circle of friends.

Gerri

While Brian framed the call we put out for help in military terms, for me it was more like that circle of life in which one set of hands reaches out to help, then another, then another. So many people Brian had helped in the past now made efforts to help him in return. It was a beautiful affirmation of the good he had done in his life and it gave me the comforting feeling that we were being buoyed along, passed along from one set of caring hands to the next.

We got Brian's diagnosis just before Memorial Day. The fact that we couldn't get in to see any doctors seemed to make that long weekend interminable. We filled the void by getting the word out; within no time, the phone was ringing off the hook. People were calling to offer sympathy and help. The help often consisted of a recommendation of "the best oncologist" or "the best neurosurgeon" around. I was amazed at how many different doctors' names were given to fit this description! It soon became apparent that in sifting through all this conflicting advice, I'd have an enormous task ahead of me.

Keep an Advocate's Notebook

Advocate Tip
#7

Before we went to our first doctor's appointment, I bought a 5-by-8 spiral notebook and began writing down names and phone numbers of doctors and appointment dates and times. When I began the journal, I had nothing more important in mind than helping myself remember names, dates, and places. The bright flowers on the cover definitely didn't broadcast professionalism on my part, so perhaps it didn't pose much of a threat to doctors when I constantly pulled it out of my purse.

Very quickly, this simple book began to evolve into a complete record of everything that was happening to Brian. On the inside front and back hard covers, I kept the phone numbers I needed to find on a regular basis. Since we would go to various cities in our effort to get the best treatment, I noted information on the ordinary things we needed while we were on the road. On the back pages, for example, I kept phone numbers for taxi companies in San Francisco, restaurants in Dallas, and an acupuncturist in Los Angeles. There were also phone numbers for various airlines and our corresponding frequent flyer numbers, and just about any information that might make life easier for us when we were traveling.

The front pages became a chronological record of Brian's appointments and what was done for (or to) him. I kept detailed notes of conversations I had with doctors or medical personnel. I wrote down information on the procedures Brian underwent. I kept records of medications he took and his reaction to them. And because we sought advice and treatment from various sources, my notebook became a record that various physicians relied on. At one point, Brian was receiving a treatment to be administered by needle. He was to be injected on one side of his body first, and in the next treatment on the other side. When no one could recall which side they had used during the last treatment, the doctor in charge of administering the injections turned to me and asked, "Gerri, what does your book say?" This really wasn't anything earthshaking or of great significance, but is an example of the importance of keeping a record.

I found that it is impossible to rely on your memory when you're on emotional overload. You are deluged with information and you need every tool available to help you get through this. Keeping a notebook or journal of everything that goes on is one of the best things an advocate can do.

That notebook is also helpful before meetings with doctors. All too often, the questions you thought of when you were at home are forgotten in the moment. Write them down in your notebook, and use it to remember everything you wanted to ask.

Now there are more complete and professional journals available for the patient or advocate. Mine was amateurish, but small enough that I could stuff it in my purse and keep it with me at all times—and it sure worked. See page 203 for a start on organizing yours.

Brian

Gerri had so much to juggle in those early days of the diagnosis, I don't know how she did it. And as if she didn't have enough on her plate, enter Brian Dennis Sean Monaghan, victim and perpetrator of 'roid rage.

Welcome to the wild world of steroid psychosis—within a few days of my diagnosis I was living it. The rapid growth of the brain tumors was causing lots of swelling in my brain, a dangerous condition that had to be controlled through the use of a heavy-duty steroid, Decadron. Twenty-four hours after I started taking it, I had become a different person. While I have the reputation of being a tough guy in the courtroom, under normal circumstances I handle life with a calm demeanor. These weren't normal circumstances. The change was dramatic. I couldn't sleep at all. I was up all night, pacing the floors and scratching at my skin. I continually ran my fingers through my hair until it stood on end—Gerri told me that I looked like Don King on a bad hair day. I started hiccuping and couldn't stop for more than twenty-four hours.

A woman of many talents, Gerri was famous for her gardenias. Normally, I loved these fragrant flowers, but one Saturday when she came into my room with a vaseful to put on the table, I found myself snarling, "You and those f—ing gardenias."

I think that by the time those words had left my mouth I knew I was in deep trouble. Gerri stormed off into the bathroom and locked the door. Within a minute I was outside that door, apologizing.

"I don't care how many brain tumors you have. That doesn't mean you can talk to me or anyone else like that," she countered.

Potential anger at your caregiver, your advocate, your family is something every patient should be aware of. I've heard many stories about people who are so angry at the stranglehold that their disease or condition has on them that they lash out at the closest person. That's usually the very same person who is right beside them, trying to take care of them.

With the exception of this first incident in which I was quickly put in my place, I didn't do that. I tried my best to keep upbeat. I knew that Gerri was doing everything she could for me, and at times, the only responsibility I had was to keep that good 'tude. So that's what I tried to do. There's a line from *Fiddler on the Roof* that I turned on its head and used as a guidepost. The beggar looks down on the one kopek now resting in the palm of his hand. He looks at the man who has given him the coin and in his heavy Yiddish accent says, "One kopek! Last time, you gave me two!" The man replies, "I had a bad day." The beggar looks back at him and says, "So you had a bad day. Why should I suffer?" 'Roid rage excepted, that's how I came to feel about getting cancer. I might be having a bad day, but that didn't mean those around me should suffer any more than they had to.

After my blowup, Gerri made some frantic calls to the doctor and he soon reduced the amount of steroids to a level that reduced the intensity of my reaction. I knew that these pills were the one lifeline I had to hang on to for now, but my extreme reaction made me totally miserable. Both Gerri and I knew that I couldn't live without the steroids, but for the first few days, neither of us was sure that I could live with them.

Advocate Tip #8

Stand Up for Yourself

It's one thing to be sympathetic to the ordeal your loved one is going through, but quite another to let an angry patient take it out on you. Brian was, with the exception of the steroid incident, a real sweetheart to me throughout his illness, but I know of other caregivers who are not treated so kindly. If your loved one is taking out his frustration on you, my advice is not to put up with it at all. It's just too much to take on. Serious illness can turn some patients into two-year-olds. If that happens, my advice is to treat them as such. Tell your patient you are willing to shoulder as much of the burden as possible, but you can't do that if he doesn't treat you well.

The steroids also had another side effect. They gave me a serious case of the "munchies." While this sounds funny, it really wasn't. This need for food was beyond anything normal, because if I didn't get food into me right away, the headaches I was experiencing on a constant basis became so intense that they almost brought me to my knees. I seemed to be hungry constantly, and Gerri began carrying around food for me in her purse. Those purses got larger and larger so that in any given instant, she could be counted on for candy bars, fruit, water, and a box of Wheat Thins.

On June 4, 1998, Gerri and I took a three-hour drive up to Santa Monica to meet with Dr. Robert Rand, a neurosurgeon at the John Wayne Cancer Institute. He turned out to be a wonderful man who took the time to explain things to us in great detail. He put my MRIs on the screen just like the doctors do on television. This was the very first time that we had seen the actual tumors in my brain. Seeing "proof" of two brain tumors was more than intimidating. Because of the contrast solution injected into my veins for help reading the MRI, the tumors looked like black holes surrounded by white halos. Melanoma brain tumors are different from other brain tumors in that they are round and perfectly spherical. The one in the occipital region (the back of the head) was about the size of a dime. The other appeared to be about the size of a quarter and was located just above my left ear.

Knowing I had tumors was one thing, but seeing those evil-looking things growing in my head was the first time that I truly felt the enormity of my medical situation. In my case, seeing was believing.

Dr. Rand was a straight shooter with a direct but kindly manner. When I insisted, he confirmed what I had already been told: that without aggressive treatment, I had only a few months to live. When I asked him to tell me how long I had if I got no treatment at all, his reply was brief and to the point. "That's kind of a moot question, Brian. Are you telling me that you're just going to ignore these tumors and not do anything?" Of course, he was right.

By the time we met with Dr. Rand, we had already learned of a procedure called Gamma Knife surgery from several other physicians. I had no idea what the hell a Gamma Knife was, and to me, it sounded like something out of a George Lucas movie. But when I learned that it meant they could get rid of the brain tumors without having to cut my head open, I thought it sounded great. Dr. Rand said that he agreed that the Gamma Knife was the best option for me. After attempting to remove the brain tumors with this technique, we would then tackle the underlying cancer itself.

Seeing those dark, dense brain tumors followed by talk of brain surgery made for a very heavy moment, but right then in Dr. Rand's office, my overriding feeling was . . . ravenous hunger. The steroid-inspired munchies took over, and in those days, the munchies ruled. I could have been having an audience with the Pope, and I would have asked him if he had any food! So in the middle of this important conference, I signaled to Gerri. Out onto the conference table came the box of Wheat Thins. In my frenzy to feed, I knocked the box over and most of the crackers spilled out onto the floor. My main focus was clearly on food, not cancer, and I think Gerri was really embarrassed. As she scrambled to pick everything up, Dr. Rand calmly brought over a paper plate and told her to put the crackers on it. When Gerri tried to throw them in the trash, he asked her to just leave them there on the conference table. Gerri looked at him quizzically, and then that uncanny intuition she often has took over. She laughed and said, "You're going to eat them, aren't you?"

Dr. Rand laughed and acknowledged that yes, indeed he was. "After years of being exposed to unbelievably bad things in an operating room, I always tell my wife that I'll eat anything off the floor with no qualms at all."

Moments of comic relief like these aside, those first two weeks after getting my diagnosis were pretty damned miserable. During that time, Gerri and I made the rounds of various doctors, medical groups, and hospitals. I was poked with countless needles, gave enough blood to start my own blood drive, and had my fill of CT scans and MRIs. In all this time, the blinding headaches never stopped, and I was still operating in a fog bank. My head just wouldn't clear and I found it difficult to focus or even think. Other than my frequent trips to the refrigerator, the only thing I wanted to do was stay in bed and sleep.

Advocate Tip #9

Get Dressed

I know this may sound like a silly suggestion, but it's something I found helpful in trying to maintain an upbeat attitude. From those very first days of dealing with this medical crisis, I had nagged Brian about one thing that he didn't want to hear. It was always along the lines of, "Get dressed. Come on, Brian. Not a jogging suit. Put on slacks and a shirt; we've got a doctor's appointment." In those early days, all he wanted to do was to stay in bed in a dark room, avoiding the outside world, and here I was, wanting him to get dressed. Groaning, he insisted that the doctors wouldn't care what he looked like; they were only interested in his brain tumors.

But I had come up with a theory, and while it took a while for Brian to agree with me, we've both decided that it was probably the right thing to do. When we walked into a crowded doctor's office, the receptionist would look at the nicely dressed couple approaching her and smile. We always seemed to get good treatment. I've told other people about this and it's made many of them angry! They feel that when it comes to getting good medical care, it shouldn't make any difference how you are clothed. And I agree. It shouldn't. But I think the reality is that it does. Maybe it's more about a positive attitude we assumed when walking into a situation, and that dressing up a little simply reflected part of that attitude. Maybe part of it is that when you act upbeat even when you feel terrible, it helps the people around you feel better about you. In turn they respond to you more quickly.

I know that there will be days when patients won't feel like getting dressed—especially when they are in great pain or recovering from an operation or fighting through chemotherapy and nausea that has them bent over the porcelain bowl. No one would expect them to pull themselves completely together then. But when they can do so, try to convince them to get dressed. It may give them a little extra edge in helping to maintain the positive attitude they so desperately need.

Looking back, this was a time of incredible uncertainty as we tried to figure out which direction to take. And I guess by we, I really mean Gerri, who was fielding input from all sides. For me, much of the time, everything was just a blur. I sort of stumbled along from one appointment to the next, my main focus on clearing the cobwebs and getting the pain to stop. Without my advocate by my side, I would have been in even worse shape.

Here's one example from those early days of how Gerri took to her new role. We were visiting a local oncologist, one of the many who came highly recommended from a friend. By now, x-rays had shown that in addition to the brain tumors, I had a small tumor near my armpit. The brain tumors posed the most immediate threat, but this metastasis in my lymph system was strong evidence that melanoma was indeed the type of cancer I had. With Gerri leading the charge, we were gathering as much information about our enemy as possible.

Gerri and I were waiting in this doctor's office to discuss our options, when in came a nurse who must have been almost as tall and hefty as I am. What's more, she was carrying a needle that looked to be about two feet long.

"I'm here to do your bone marrow biopsy," she said matter-of-factly.

Sitting on an exam table in the doctor's office, the flimsy paper rustling under me, I couldn't take my eyes off the enormous needle the nurse held in her hand. The woman towered over me. I looked to Gerri, who was sitting in the corner.

"What's that for?" Gerri asked. "Why does he have to have a bone marrow biopsy?"

The nurse replied she didn't know why, but she did know that the doctor had sent her into the room to do it, and that's what she was going to do.

"This doesn't make any sense to me," Gerri went on. "I'd like to talk to the doctor before you do this. Would you please ask him to come in here?"

Then it started. In an angry voice, the nurse insisted that she had been sent in by a very busy doctor to do a job, that she was a very experienced nurse, that she knew what she was doing, and that she intended to do what she had been sent in to do.

Gerri stepped between me and Nurse Ratched.

"You're not touching him! Now, go get the doctor."

As the nurse stormed out, it occurred to me that the woman was probably right. She probably did know what she was doing and she was obviously pissed that her authority had been questioned. I had the feeling that when she got back, she was probably going to shove that long needle up my ass! At any rate, it wasn't going to be pretty.

A few minutes later, the doctor came in, closed the door, and leaned back against it, very embarrassed. Sheepishly, he said, "I'm sorry. That needle was not intended for you. It was for somebody else. I apologize."

It turns out that this procedure, while extremely painful, would not have caused me any permanent damage, but that's not the point. It's an example of the need for an advocate, the need to have someone other than the patient question what's being done and why. You need someone to stand up for you when something doesn't sound right, someone who is not intimidated by the fact that the person standing in front of her is wearing a white coat.

You can be a lawyer, a scientist, a teacher, even a doctor, but when you are the patient in a critical situation, you desperately need an advocate. I think that in many ways, you as a patient have got to put your faith in the medical profession. As a lawyer, I always wanted my clients to put their faith in me and in the decisions I was making for them. That's not to say that I never screwed up, but they needed to believe that I was in charge and knew what was best. Now, I needed to believe whatever the people in white coats told me. If they said bend over for this shot, I was ready to do it. I had faith in them. I really think that you need to believe in them.

But while I needed to believe, Gerri didn't. This is where that need for an advocate standing by your side to ask questions is vital. There was no doubt in my mind that Gerri was handling everything now. She had been my wife and my best friend, and now she stepped into her new role with great strength. I don't know how she did it, but somehow she was able not only to protect me from nurses with big needles, but to sort through all the information and advice we were being given.

Gerri

I spent those first few days after Brian's diagnosis making and receiving phone calls, meeting with local doctors, and doing more research than I'd ever done as a paralegal.

Brian and I were both whiz kids at playing solitaire on the computer, but in May of 1998, anything much beyond that was out of reach for us. Our ability to do any computer research was virtually nonexistent. I knew that there had to be information available on the computer, but where did I start? I needed help and so I did what has become a staple for me in fighting this battle. I asked for help. Within a short time, my son Mark and his wife, Sharon, had responded and were churning out lists of websites for me—and of even greater importance, they were teaching me how to use them. I couldn't have done it without them. I'm not sure where Mark and Sharon started their research back in 1998, but I know that when they typed in the words "gamma knife surgery," it was enough to provide us with mounds of information on that procedure.

Within a few hours, I was reading articles and looking at photos that showed me what the Gamma Knife looked like. For the first time, I learned that it really was not surgery in the traditional sense but instead a procedure that used gamma radiation to effectively kill off the brain tumors by altering their ability to reproduce. This was the first real ray of hope we had for Brian and there it was, right on the Internet.

A few weeks into our odyssey, we were fortunate enough to find a local oncologist, Dr. Bob Brouillard, who was willing to help us step outside the box in our search for the right treatment plan for Brian. In fact, Dr. Brouillard was the person who told us that no one oncologist can possibly know all the various treatments available for the dozens of different types of cancer. Most relevant to our case, the National Comprehensive Cancer Network (NCCN), a nonprofit alliance of some of the world's leading cancer centers, has established a series of treatment plans or guidelines for various types of cancer. The guidelines offered by these experts might contain a treatment that your doctor just isn't aware of. No matter what your disease, researching treatment plans is one of the best things you can do for your patient. (The NCCN is allied with the American Cancer Society—see page 211 for details.)

As an advocate, it's your responsibility to find as much information as you can, and without hesitation, bring that information to your local doctor. You're fighting for your patient's life, so go online, get as much information as you can, and give it to your doctor.

Make Use of the Internet

We are all so fortunate that we live in this age of the Internet. It's a wonderful source of information, and although some physicians are apoplectic at the fact that a layperson could possess enough information to question his or her sacrosanct physician-only knowledge, we've found that the really competent physicians are not threatened by a patient or advocate who is willing to learn more about a disease. In your search for answers, you may want to start just by logging on to a search engine like Google and typing in a specific illness, treatment, or surgical procedure. You will then be led to more specific sites, the best of which are created by medical professionals. In response to the increased ability to use the computer for research, many other websites are now available that will provide this same type of information, among them www.medlineplus .org, a site run by the National Institutes of Health.

My words of caution on using the Internet to do your research are pretty simple. First, with the rapid changes and advancements in the medical field, make sure that the article you're looking at is current. Then, look at whether the websites are from governmental agencies (such as the NIH), nonprofits (a university or medical center), or for-profits (such as WebMD). All three have good information, but you need to know where their bias might be in recommending a type of treatment.

Remember, the best website in the world is not a physician. You can bring your doctor the information you've obtained; you can raise questions based on information you've gleaned off a website; but in the end, neither you nor a website has the medical knowledge of a professional. That said, the Internet is a great weapon to have at your disposal in this battle, and you'll need every weapon available. So don't be intimidated.

What if you barely know how to get online? Those of us who are "older" are probably fortunate enough to have younger people in our family who see the Internet as an essential part of life. Ask them for help. Chances are they'll be happy to do some of the legwork for you. Even if you have to go outside your family, do it. And if other people offer to help, take them up on it. It's a win-win for everyone.

It quickly became apparent that other than the Gamma Knife, which sounded hopeful, the rest of the information coming my way was very negative. Many friends were reaching out to people they knew in the medical community, but the words coming back to me were always, "Gerri, it doesn't look good." Friends inundated us with calls and recommendations in their very best attempts to help. As I tried to understand one course of action, I found that the very next one might be in complete opposition. I felt whipsawed.

This time was very difficult for me. I worked hard at staying positive in hopes that I could keep Brian positive, too. I was determined not to let him see my doubts and fears.

Our call to general quarters went far and wide, and for me in those early days, it also meant calling on God. I know that Brian didn't feel the need for formal religion at this point, but I did. After several years away from church, that very first Sunday after the diagnosis, I was back. I was willing to do any novena, say any prayer, rub on any holy oil, or make any promise necessary to keep him alive.

Brian

As a young Irish Catholic kid in Philadelphia I was very religious. Every time I wrote anything on paper, certainly when writing an answer to a test question, at the very top of each page I wrote "JMJ" (which of course means "Jesus, Mary, and Joseph"). It was done with the hope that they would provide me with some much-needed assistance, if not the specific answers to the test questions. When I played sports, particularly basketball, God must have been worn out from trying to help me with my lousy jump shots. Imagine, if you would, that I've launched the ball into the air. Like most of my shots, it will never get close to the basket. Nevertheless, I've asked God to drop that ball cleanly through the net. By the way, if God had dropped it in (which was really the only way it was ever going to get there when the ball had come from my hands), everyone in the place would have known that they had witnessed a miracle to rival the loaves and fishes. It was a lot to ask of God, and I'm sure He had much more important things on his plate than my basketball game.

When my illness struck, in addition to Gerri's prayers, numerous prayer circles, novenas, and rosaries were said on my behalf and I welcomed every one of them. I was happy to take any help I could get, so although I didn't reach out for God's intervention on my own, I had scores of friends and family members who did that for me. Or in some cases, with me. On one occasion, a caring and very religious friend came over with guitar in hand and prayed for me in song. When I went to the hospital, priests would appear at my bedside to visit and pray. I was happy with it all, as I figured all these people might well be in a better position than I was to bargain with God.

Address the Question of Faith

Advocate Tip
#**11**

At some point in your loved one's illness, early on or not, questions about faith will arise. Maybe he or she will suffer a crisis of faith, maybe "find religion," or maybe, as in Brian's case, not change his own beliefs at all but develop more of an appreciation for those who do have a strong faith and want to share it. For you, their advocate, these questions may arise, too.

My advice is to be open to whatever you and your patient are feeling when it comes to faith, and know that in times of serious illness, ideas about faith may shift and change.

Gerri

Initially Brian's headaches were what he characterized as blinding, and for a while he was unable to do much more than sleep. The fog he was living in didn't allow for much thinking, so much of the decision making was up to me. Coming up with a course of action that would be the best for Brian was a heavy responsibility, and although I had a lot of good input and encouragement from several friends as well as my sons, I knew that in the end, the big decisions were left to me.

During those first few weeks, one thought kept me in a constant state of terror: yes, we'd have to deal with the cancer that had metastasized in Brian's body, but inside his head were two brain tumors that were growing rapidly. The doctors told me that the tumors had caused a great deal of swelling of the surrounding brain tissue, and that this swelling was causing the headaches and the mixing up of words and his not being able to remember things. The steroids he had started would begin to control the swelling, but only for so long. Time was not on our side.

We had to deal with these brain tumors first; later on, we could begin to deal with the cancer itself. But I needed to take the time necessary to find out just what was the best medical route for Brian, then we needed to decide what doctors and medical facilities we wanted to use. And all this had to be accomplished in as little time as possible.

Balancing the need for action with the need to take your time and make a good decision can be such a difficult line to walk. If it's at all possible, I urge you to take some time and, again, follow your instincts.

Within those first few weeks, one of the doctors we saw recommended "a light dusting of whole-brain radiation." It has such a benign ring to it, doesn't it? I must have remembered the old jokes about putting your head in a microwave oven, because I asked him, "Wouldn't there be problems for Brian?" His reply was that *if* Brian lived "long term," he would indeed suffer significant "cognitive deficits." I insisted on an explanation in layman's terms, and when pressed, the doctor defined "long term" as eighteen months to two years, and "cognitive deficits" as, well, "cognitive deficits."

In short, he was telling me that my husband was unlikely to be alive in two years and that if he was, his mental functions would be hugely compromised. In the past, we had both talked about not wanting to live in a condition where we were severely mentally impaired. Especially after watching his brother Terry's decline, Brian had made it clear that he would not want this option. Instantly, I knew that this wasn't where we needed to be for his medical treatment. It was obvious that it was time to move on.

By contrast, when we met with Dr. Rand, he agreed with the recommendation we had already received that Brian have Gamma Knife surgery to deal with the brain tumors. I asked him, "If you had this condition, where would you go?" He replied that he would head straight for one of the major brain tumor centers in California, and that he was personally comfortable in recommending either Good Samaritan in Los Angeles or the University of California, San Francisco Medical Center. His reason was one that struck a chord with both of us. Dr. Rand told us that these two medical centers utilized a team approach. They had several highly regarded neurosurgeons who worked on a daily basis both with doctors who were radiation oncologists and also with physicists who did the number crunching on where to aim the gamma rays that would be going into Brian's skull to—in his words—"zap those suckers." That's Brian Monaghan–speak for destroy the brain tumors!

The idea of a team approach really made sense to Brian and to me.

Brian

Maybe it's my old sports background or my schooling at the Naval Academy, but I've found that anytime you work together as a team, you work better. It was the same concept I had tried to use in my years of trial practice. I did my best to make sure that the people who worked in my office knew I couldn't win any case without them. Whether I was talking to Joyce, the best word processor ever, or Carre, the receptionist who fielded all calls, I did my best to make sure they understood we were a team. Now that concept really resonated with me. I wanted to be in the hands of people who worked together on a constant basis. I wanted a team where everyone was on the same page, all of the time.

Find Physicians with a Team Approach

Many doctors pay lip service to working as a team, but that doesn't mean they do. When you're gathering information from various physicians, ask them if they utilize a team approach. A true team approach means that the same group of people—surgeons, anesthesiologists, nurses—consistently work together in providing treatment and handling procedures for their patients. For this reason, they are not only highly skilled, but practiced and comfortable supporting one another to achieve the task at hand.

Gerri

In these early weeks of visiting numerous doctors and exploring myriad treatment options, my learning curve for how to be an advocate was steep. As we trucked from appointment to appointment, I was learning about how to take Brian's health into our own hands as we searched for the right doctors and facilities.

That battle plan I had written the night of the diagnosis, the one with the broad categories—research, physicians, nutrition, communication network—and names next to them, had been a good place to start. Now I was putting the plan into action, filling in each category with more and more information.

For example, on the research front I was asking the fundamental question, What is this disease, melanoma? At first, I only knew that it was our enemy, but I needed to know more about it in order to beat it. Having sat next to Brian on numerous occasions as he watched *Patton*, I now remembered a scene from the movie that seemed vitally important to me. The army is in Africa and General Patton has just outsmarted German Field Marshal Rommel. Patton squints into his binoculars and then says, "Rommel, you magnificent bastard, I read your book."

While I didn't think of melanoma as magnificent in any sense of the word, I understood that I needed to "read the book" on it and learn everything I could.

Physicians and ideas about nutrition were fast being added to the initial plan. As for the communication network, handling that was a big part of what I was doing at this time.

I asked the question, Whom do we know who can help? We were fortunate in knowing people with contacts in the medical world, and that certainly helped facilitate our search for answers. But by putting Brian's call to general quarters into action, the word spread out beyond our normal circle of friends, to as many people as possible—old college friends, neighbors, friends of friends. You never know where that ripple effect can lead. It could be that the sweet eighty-year-old lady who lives across the street just might have a grandson, now living in Chicago, who has just developed the very latest cutting-edge research on your particular disease. Of course, sweet Mrs. Smith would be happy to call him, and of course, he will later take your call. First, it's his grandmother who called, and second, he's looking for volunteers for his clinical trial and your patient might just be the perfect candidate. But none of it will happen if you don't get the word out! You need help from every and any corner imaginable. Let the people at your church know. Ask your family to spread the word at their churches. Let the teachers at the local schools know. Call the colleges and universities in your city and find out if anyone knows of anyone doing research in the relevant medical field.

You will find that friends and family will be more than happy to help. They often *need* to help, so don't turn them down. If you're filled with such an abundance of pride that it makes it difficult for you to ask for help, remember: this is not about you. You are the advocate, not the patient. The beneficiary of this help is your loved one.

Let me share something else, something you may find painful, as I did. You will find some family and friends who can't help you or won't, and you may never know the reason for this. Perhaps they simply can't deal with the thought of losing their father or mother or brother or friend, and they become paralyzed by that fear. Whatever the reason, you are going to be disappointed by some people you thought you could count on. My advice to you is to move on and not dwell on it. You can sort out those relationships and disappointments later. Right now, you need to harness your energy into fighting this disease. Don't waste it being upset with others. Besides, you'll find that someone else will step up to the plate, someone you had not counted on, but who came through for you just when you needed him or her most.

Put the Battle Plan into Action

Research: As an advocate, you always need to keep updating your knowledge of your patient's disease, and writing down questions you have for the doctors.

Physicians: All doctors are not equal, and not every one is right for your patient. Continue to explore as many possibilities as you can, and go with people you feel good about.

Nutrition: Use the Internet and advice of doctors to find out how you can support your patient's immune system and general health through this difficult time.

Communication Network: Update your list of everyone you know who might be able to help, and don't be afraid to share with them what's going on. Don't fret over people you thought might do more, and be prepared to accept help from unlikely quarters.

Brian

Overall, in the first weeks after the diagnosis, our approach was to reach out to everyone we knew or could think of who might be able to help gather information or offer contacts. Too often in the past, people ran from the word "cancer." I'm old enough to remember a time when no one would even say it. Instead, they spoke in hushed voices about "the big C." I think that's an attitude long past its time, not worth following, and I'll tell you why.

It was because a friend, John Lynch, heard about my diagnosis that he contacted one of his friends, Donna Rosen, who volunteered as the head of the auxiliary at the John Wayne Cancer Center. It was Donna Rosen who would immediately get me the appointment there with Dr. Rand. When my client Tom Self got word of my diagnosis, he contacted a former classmate who now heads up the M. D. Anderson Cancer Center, who in turn arranged for me to be seen within days. When my old friend Sol Price heard of the diagnosis, he contacted Dr. Charlie Wilson, head of neurosurgery at University of California, San Francisco Medical Center. Years ago, Dr. Wilson had helped care for Sol's grandson Aaron, and now he made time to see me.

Issue a Call to General Quarters

Advocate Tip
#14

We understand that not everybody has access to the sort of network we had. However, that doesn't mean that you and your patient shouldn't put out the news of the diagnosis. Your cousin's cousin might know somebody from high school who's now doing research at a medical lab. Your coworker's aunt might have had the same condition as your patient, and been successfully treated at a medical center in another city. In other words, don't think you don't know anybody who can help. You do.

There are many more examples of one hand after another reaching out to help me. Gerri and I sure as hell didn't do this on our own. I'm firmly convinced that if the call to general quarters hadn't gone out, we would have been limited in our choices. Getting cancer—or for that matter, any other life-threatening disease—is not something you caused. So don't take sole responsibility for it. Don't hide from cancer. Say it out loud: "I've got cancer." Now, damn it, do something about it. Reach out to everyone you know. Let them reach out to the people they know. Draw on every resource you have, every resource they have. Send out that call to general quarters.

Gerri

In those early weeks after the diagnosis, our research had us leaning toward having the Gamma Knife surgery in Los Angeles. But we still wanted to be sure that we were making the best decision possible based on the great leads we were getting from all over.

That meant one more big trip.

Chapter Four

REVEL IN LAUGHTER AND THE LOVE OF FRIENDS

From quiet homes and first beginning,
Out to the undiscovered ends,
There's nothing worth the wear of winning,
But laughter and the love of friends.

—HILAIRE BELLOC

Brian

At 9:00 a.m., the glass doors of the M. D. Anderson Cancer Center in Houston, Texas, slid open for us. As we crossed the large hotel-like lobby, we were approached by two women wearing white jackets and carrying clipboards. In a heavy Texas accent, one of them greeted us: "I bet y'all are the Monaghans from San Diego. We're here to show y'all around so you don't get lost."

M. D. Anderson is one of the most renowned cancer centers in the world. As we followed our guides through the clean, ultramodern hallways, I thought about how getting here was the result of the calls made on our behalf by our friend Tom Self. His contact, a former classmate from medical school, had greased the wheels of this institution, and here Gerri and I were being welcomed with warm Texas hospitality. The staff couldn't have been nicer.

We were immediately shown into the office of their melanoma specialist. We shook hands, made introductions all around, and began the usual chatter. But as we were talking, the doctor kept looking at me with a quizzical expression. Suddenly, he seemed to have one of those "aha!" moments. "I have seen you before," he said.

"I don't think so, doctor. We got here late last night and I've never been to Houston before. I don't think we've ever met."

He was adamant. "I have seen you. When I was shaving. I saw you on *The Today Show*!"

You can call it what you want: the luck of the Irish, a twist of fate—whatever. But here it was again. It turned out that he had seen me on TV the day before while he was shaving. When the Self trial had ended back in April, I had been interviewed about the impact of the case on managed care. While *I* thought it was a huge case (that's pronounced "yooge" in the Philly way, with a silent "h"), *The Today Show* obviously didn't think it was earth shattering, so they aired it on a slow news day. We'd had no idea when it would air, so initially we had no idea what the doctor was talking about.

Although lawyers are not always the most popular people in the medical world, this time it was different. As the doctor said, "You have done something wonderful for medicine and for doctors." He briefly stepped out of the room and called in a neurosurgeon, who had also seen the same program. For a few minutes, we all cheerfully discussed the benefits our trial results might have. It was a very warm and happy moment.

It went rapidly downhill from there.

We asked for the truth about my situation and they gave it to us. Their recommendations were different from everything else we had heard to date. They told us they didn't believe the Gamma Knife would be effective in dealing with the brain tumors, and they strongly recommended immediate brain surgery. In fact, the neurosurgeon said that he would rearrange his schedule so that the craniotomy could be done the following day. I knew that he was making a valid point—one argument for neurosurgery was that it would have a more immediate effect on getting rid of the tumors than the Gamma Knife, which would mean I could get off the damned steroids sooner. That part sounded good, but having my head carved open as opposed to the noninvasive Gamma Knife? No thanks.

The bad news just kept getting worse. As kindly as he could, their oncologist told us that the only method proven to have any success at all against metastatic melanoma was a potent combination of chemotherapy with some interferon thrown in for good measure. He told us that the drug combination they planned to use would result in infamous side effects: high fever, chills, general malaise, mouth sores, loss of hair, frequent bleeding, and frequent infections. The IV chemo dosage would be so high that it would be necessary for me to be hospitalized while I took it. On top of it all, the treatment would take eleven months, so I would have to move from San Diego to Houston.

I think of myself as a pretty tough guy, and while the prospect of going through brain surgery followed by eleven months of chemotherapy didn't make me happy, I knew that I could handle anything if I had to. You can deal with whatever comes your way if you have an end game in mind. But this end game didn't look so good. When we pressed them for some statistic we could hang our hopes on, the doctors didn't give us much encouragement. They told me that my life during the eleven months of treatment would be a living hell. When I asked how that ordeal would improve my chances of survival, they said they hoped that after the treatment, they could give me perhaps another year of life. But, they cautioned, in melanoma patients without the complication of brain tumors, only 15 percent had their cancer "under control" two years out.

One look between Gerri and me was all we needed. Gerri's initial research had led her to believe that this more "standard" treatment had a very limited chance of success. She had already started to talk about the need for us to push the envelope. I didn't need much convincing. The whole idea of being aggressive and "going for it" was the way I had lived my life. It was a philosophy that had always worked for me, and I didn't think that this was the time to change. I know that some people are only willing to accept the tried and true. But I could see only the "tried" part in this scenario, and it didn't ring true. This was neurosurgery and toxic chemotherapy and everything we had been told didn't work. Plus, it was eleven months in Houston away from my home, family, and friends, and to me that sounded like a death sentence right there.

It was a terribly dark moment for me. But what makes me laugh now is the memory of Gerri turning to the doctor and telling him that we had to leave right then to catch a plane. He sputtered and said, "Why, I haven't even examined your husband yet." She told him that he had about ten minutes while she brought the car around. Then I watched as Gerri and a nurse got into a tug-of-war over my CT scans. Literally, a tug-of-war. The nurse held on to them, insisting that since she had already checked them into their system, the scans now belonged to them. Gerri explained otherwise, and soon the scans were back in our control.

Get Copies of Records

In the past, medical charts were easier to sneak a peek at since they were at least hard copies, but now they're often stored on computers. It's important to know that this is information you can request, so ask to see the doctor's orders. If nothing else, it shows the staff that you're paying attention. Remember, these are your records—or rather, the patient's records. With recent rules in place that make it much more difficult for anyone to get access to medical records, you, as an advocate, may be told that you don't have the right to look at them. You do! Ask for a release form and have your patient sign it, stating that you are authorized to have access to the records. *Don't* buy into the false idea that these records belong to the hospital or the medical provider. If you are hesitant to believe this, just remember that doctors' offices and hospitals allow your insurance carrier access to your records. You want the same access, and don't be afraid to say so.

As a valuable diagnostic tool, doctors often order MRIs and CT scans. Don't settle for a written report of the scan's results. Ask for a duplicate set of the scans themselves. This is especially important in the early stages of the diagnosis process when, hopefully, you will be seeking a second opinion. No doctor wants to simply rely on a report written by someone else. They will want to review the scans themselves. So when those scans are being done, go up to the receptionist and simply ask that a second set be made. Think of it as ordering a duplicate set of photos. In fact, in the ten years since Brian's diagnosis, medical technology has improved to such a degree that our recent follow-up scans are put onto a CD, which is then sent to our physicians for review. Even if you're charged for the disk or the films themselves, the charge is minimal, especially when compared to having to go through another round of scans within a few days.

With sincere thanks to everyone at M. D. Anderson for all their warmth and hospitality, we were out of there. Once again, it was time to move on. Our hope was that we would somehow move forward. For now, all we knew was that we would have to continue our search for the best answers.

Emotionally, Gerri and I reached the absolute low point. We recognized that unless something drastic happened, I had only months to live. Before arriving in Houston, we had been very excited about the Gamma Knife as a solution for dealing with the brain tumors. Now we'd been told that it wouldn't work. We had previously been told that chemo had a terrible track record in curing melanoma, and now we had been told that it was the best recommendation these experts had. During the drive back to the airport, Gerri just keep reaching over and squeezing my hand. Neither one of us was capable of saying much.

We had hitched a ride to Houston with John Moores in his private jet. John, a man known not only as the owner of the San Diego Padres, but also for his big heart and major philanthropic work, had heard that we were headed to Houston to seek a second opinion. He had called and told us he was flying there on business, and if the dates worked out he'd be happy to take us along.

By the time we were ready to leave Houston, I was mentally and physically exhausted and truly down. And I probably looked it. Early in the flight, John suggested that I stretch out on the sofa and get some sleep. I remember insisting that I was fine but he would have none of it and instead told me, "Lie down, buddy. Better men than you have slept on this sofa." John wrapped both Gerri and me in the warmth of blankets and friendship on the plane trip home. A simple act of kindness—yet it helped cut through the gloom that had enveloped us.

Bum a Ride

Advocate Tip
#16

Offering a ride in his private plane was a kind gesture, but it turns out that John Moores is not alone in doing this. We have since learned that individual pilots and even corporations will often offer to transport patients of all types, not just cancer victims, free of charge. If you have a life-threatening illness and need to travel to another city for treatment, there are several organizations that provide flights in small jets for no cost. See page 212 for a contact list.

Gerri

This was clearly a low point for us both. We had heard such great things about M. D. Anderson, and for so many patients, it's considered a mecca for cancer treatment. I know that its reputation is well deserved, but it just wasn't the right place to pursue Brian's treatment.

Not only did the option of chemo and craniotomy not appeal to us given the low potential payoff, but Brian is such a social animal that he really needed the companionship of friends and family. Being isolated in Houston, or anyplace else for that matter, would have had a demoralizing effect on him, and while he could put up with anything in order to achieve a good result, this treatment plan didn't hold out much of a future for him.

When we got to the airport, before boarding the plane, I found a quiet spot for Brian to stretch out and he immediately fell into an exhausted sleep. I am usually pretty stoical, but now the pain came flooding out. I held up a magazine to give myself some cover, but as I sat there, tears were streaming down my face. Who knows what the people around me thought I was going through. Inside, I was really struggling with what the doctors had described, albeit in very kind terms, as a pretty hopeless situation. Our idea of pushing the envelope seemed to be little more than a pipe dream. I sat there trying to convince myself that we had only been on this search for about two weeks, and we weren't about to throw in the towel yet. Still, right then, things seemed pretty hopeless.

Brian

To say our experience at M. D. Anderson felt like a slug in the stomach is an understatement. What helped me get past it was, again, a circle of friends who were no strangers to tragedy.

In November 1989, a well-loved local San Diego attorney, Dan Broderick, and his new bride, Linda, were murdered in their bed by Dan's former wife, who snuck into their home before dawn and shot them both at point-blank range. The loss of Dan and Linda was incredibly hard for their many friends, but what came out of it made the healing process even more significant.

In 1991, fourteen of Dan and Linda's close friends and family began a journey together that would not only help bring us some closure, but would create a tight circle of friends. It's a circle that I think will remain together until the last of us is left. That September, the group traveled to Ireland so we could bury Dan and Linda's ashes there. More than half were lawyers (many in different specialties), while the rest were successful businessmen. Not a shy, retiring wallflower in the group.

For two weeks, we traveled together across Ireland singing, drinking, laughing, crying, and in an all-too-typical man style, mocking each other. There was a shared sense that our mission was to honor Dan and Linda. What was special about this group was the fact that each of us was a very powerful individual, and yet, in these circumstances, everyone gave each other the space to say whatever he needed to say, to recite his favorite poem, to sing his favorite song, to express his own thoughts. It was really an extraordinary collection of people and I had never seen anything like this before. It was as though the death of these good friends allowed each of us the freedom to step back from our egos and give each other respect and space.

Close to midnight of our last night in Ireland, we left our pub in Doolin—just north of the Cliffs of Moher—and walked out to the cliff, and dug a hole to bury their ashes. It was a night that I will never forget. There was love. There was sadness. We had each lost Dan and Linda, but by the end of those two weeks in Ireland, we had each gained something special. We grew to love one another in a way that was more powerful than sports teammates. We have become known as The Lads.

Upon our return to the States, we vowed that as a group we would go back to Ireland every three years and continue to remain friends. We have done so. But we do more than just drink, laugh, sing, and have fun together. We are there for each other whenever help is needed. Like the general population at large, our group has gone through its battles. Several members have battled cancer or suffered heart attacks. We lost one of the best of The Lads, Bob MacNamara, to colon cancer.

I know that we've often been characterized as wild men, and we have downed a pint or two in celebration of many things. But I find that as we have gotten older, the celebrations usually center around our love and respect for each other.

It was this group that I met up with upon my return from M. D. Anderson.

In an effort to show their support, The Lads had set up a welcome home gathering at Reidy O'Neil's, our favorite watering hole. Since several of these men are lawyers who represent doctors, they'd put out numerous calls asking for medical opinions on my chances for recovery. No one had given them any good news and by the time we gathered, the word had been passed among them that the prognosis was six months to a year at best. Although I was looking forward to seeing The Lads, I had in no uncertain terms told the main organizers,

Ed Chapin and Mike Neil, that I did not want a sobby, melancholy get-together. I think that men often deal with difficult times by trying to "tough" their way through, and with the help of song, laughter, and some Bushmills or Guinness, the Irish are masters at this. Ed and Mike passed along the word that I would be there, but only if everybody understood that there were to be no tears. The deal was, as we said in the navy, no PDAs (public displays of affection).

As Gerri and I pulled up curbside, the first thing I saw was my good friend, Ed Chapin, who at 6 feet 5 inches is a giant of a man. A giant, but a big softy, too. Ed stood there, tears streaming down his face. The idea of no display of emotion was shot!

Somehow we got through that and went on into the room where the rest of the group was gathered. There were lots of handshakes and lots of hugs. Not the kind you usually see among men, when we wear that pained expression that says, "Don't get *too* close." No. These were big, warm-hearted, full-on hugs, punctuated by big slaps on the back.

For little more than an hour, there was drinking, the singing of Irish songs, and an overarching sense of false bravado. I didn't know it at the time, but a day or two before, many of these same men had gathered together, Catholic and non-Catholic alike, at a nearby church to say a rosary on my behalf (I imagine some of them must have gone in disguise in hopes that their prayers might have more value!). If I had known that this lumbering group of drinking buddies had all knelt together and prayed for me, I think I would have been the one with tears running down my face.

After our harrowing experience in Houston, spending an hour surrounded by good, caring friends was an enormous lift for my spirits. We should all do this every day, no matter what our circumstances. But when you're in a battle like I was, being surrounded by your band of brothers (or sisters) can make it easier to get through the most intolerable days. I know that by itself, the idea of laughter and the love of friends can't keep you alive. But it sure as hell can make life worth living.

Get Your Patient Together with Friends

Brian never needs an excuse to gather with friends, and being sick didn't change this. But some patients we know do tend to retreat from the very company that can do their spirits so much good. In your role as an advocate, make some calls to friends, alerting them to the fact that your loved one could use a visit. Lunch, a long walk, or a round of golf can be a wonderful mood lifter. It's possible that the patient may initially turn down an invitation from these friends, so give them some ammunition, as in, "Don't you think your advocate could use a break? Let's get you out of the house for a while."

For those advocates whose patients aren't able to get out and about, but who have access to a computer, there is a great website, www.caringbridge.org, that allows you to post journal entries so family and friends can share your journey as they read your medical diary. Although this approach was not for me, I know of others who found it cathartic and rewarding. You can go into as much or as little detail as you wish, and for the patient, it's a way to receive get-well thoughts and prayers from friends and family who are unable to visit.

Over the years, I had developed a close friendship with Sol Price, who had been a witness for a client of mine. Because Sol was the founder of the Price Club, which later merged with Costco, he was considered by many to be the "father of discount merchandising," a title he dislikes. (His infamous response to that title is, "If that's true, I should have used a condom.") When I got my diagnosis, he was one of the first people Gerri contacted. Despite his reputation for crustiness, Sol immediately went to work on my behalf.

Sadly, he had a base of information upon which he could draw: about ten years earlier, his grandson Aaron Price had died of brain tumors. Aaron had received the best treatment available from the doctors at the University of California, San Francisco Medical Center, but despite this, he had lost his battle. As Sol often said, "Sometimes all the money in the world can't make things right." Despite that awful loss, Sol believed that the medical care at UCSF was top-notch and the doctors, especially their world-renowned neurosurgeon Dr. Charlie Wilson, were the best around.

The day after we returned from Houston, Sol called to say that he had set up a meeting for us in San Francisco with the doctors at UCSF. By this time, Gerri and I had already made the decision that despite the negative reports we had received in Houston, we were going to have Gamma Knife surgery at Good Samaritan Hospital in Los Angeles, a respected facility closer to home.

Gerri

When Sol Price calls, people listen. And that includes us. Brian and I had already decided on having the Gamma Knife done up in Los Angeles. I was exhausted from exploring options and relieved to have a clear course of action set, however much of a pipe dream it might be. But after Sol's call, we decided that out of our great respect for him and his intense involvement in our search for help, we'd go up to San Francisco and get a "second" second opinion.

Advocate Tip #18

Get a Second—or Even Third—Opinion

Brian and I are always amazed at the number of people who will accept as gospel the recommendations of one physician. If you have a brain aneurism or a heart attack or something that is immediately life threatening, you don't have a choice. You have to accept what you're told and hope and pray that you're dealing with someone who really knows what he or she is talking about. But if your situation is not immediately life threatening, by all means get a second opinion.

Don't get one from within the same medical group, or even at the same hospital. If possible, try to get an opinion from physicians in another city. We have found that doctors who practice in the same city often think alike or follow the same procedures. Getting an opinion from outside the same medical culture can give you more options.

People have given us many reasons as to why they don't seek a second opinion, but most simply don't hold water. Some have told us that they "don't want to offend" the first doctor. "What if I decide on the first doctor after all? Won't he or she be angry with me, resent me, and not give me good care?" Our answer to this is, not at all. Not if the doctor is any good.

The team of doctors we assembled and were lucky enough to have in our corner were all so competent, all so confident, and all so capable of working within their egos, that they were open to both questions and second opinions. If your physician is not, ask yourself if it's because that doctor is insecure in what he or she is telling you. And if that's the case, is this the doctor you want taking care of your patient?

We know individuals who were reluctant to get a second opinion because the first one sounded so logical that they assumed the doctor had all the information and knowledge that was needed. It may well be the case, but whenever I hear that as an excuse to not get a second opinion, I always ask: Did you buy the first car you looked at and pay the price quoted just because it looked good and the price sounded reasonable? Did you buy the first house you looked at or did you look at other homes on the market? Did you buy the first dress you saw or did you at least look at others? Do you try on only one pair of shoes before buying them?

How could you do less when it comes to a decision that could affect whether or not your patient lives or dies? Or walks or talks? How could you *not* get a second opinion?

I'm usually pretty cool, calm, and collected. But right now I was operating on emotional overload. Even with my trusty notebook in hand, I recognized how easy it was to misunderstand or misinterpret information I was hearing. I thought I'd like another set of ears to help me listen, so I invited our friend Ginny Nelson on the trip to San Francisco. Her wide range of medical knowledge was bound to provide good insight. My son Todd and his wife, Jennifer, had flown in from Denver to offer some moral support, and when he offered to be our driver, I welcomed having his shoulder to lean on.

So off we went. I don't believe that we even brought along any luggage. It was just going to be a day trip.

While the building complex at M. D. Anderson was beautiful, pristine, and even serene, UCSF was anything but. Somewhere in the world, there's a warehouse containing vats and vats of paint left over from WWII. The paint comes in just a few colors: mustard yellow, a dull rosy pink, a war-weary green, and a joyless blue, all colors designed to depress the spirit. Apparently, those vats of paint are only allowed to be distributed to large institutions like the Army, VA hospitals, old schools, your local Department of Motor Vehicles, and university hospitals. They typify what many parts of UCSF looked like, and it wasn't pretty. The buildings were old and teeming with people rushing about in every direction. We proceeded down long, bleak, narrow corridors—it was not a great start.

But then the people power of UCSF took over.

Our first meeting was with Dr. William Wara, a radiation oncologist. Brian, Ginny, Todd, and I crowded around Dr. Wara in a very tiny exam room, and I explained Brian's problem and the medical odyssey we'd been on. Then I began asking him about our options. I clearly remember that I asked Dr. Wara about the concept one doctor had put forward of "whole brain radiation."

He responded, "I don't think any sentient human being would want that." He smiled and said he believed that description covered everyone in the room. Those words alone began to overcome the depressing surroundings of this old facility. We had been more or less sure that we were going to Los Angeles for the Gamma Knife treatment—it was only a two-hour drive from our house and the facility had a great reputation. But now I had my first inkling that there was another place to consider.*

*For Todd Wortmann's perspective on how we trusted our instincts, see page 206.

Brian

After the meeting with Dr. Wara, we spent some time with Dr. Charlie Wilson. Although small in stature he is a giant in his field, and the contact that Sol had made with him meant he opened doors for us that may have taken days to do otherwise. Gerri and I sat in his office, and with great calm and confidence, Dr. Wilson told us that he thought that the Gamma Knife was the best way to go, and that UCSF was the place to have it done. We learned that UCSF had done over 600 Gamma Knife procedures in the past year alone, and that unlike several of the other facilities we had explored, they operated as a team. The team approach (they even had dedicated neuro-anesthesiologists) was definitely a huge plus for us, and the quiet confidence Dr. Wilson and everyone else there exhibited gave me the feeling that this was where I belonged.

It wasn't long into the meeting with Dr. Wilson that I turned to Gerri and said, "Let's do it!" She didn't hesitate for a moment before agreeing. Dr. Wilson juggled some schedules around and really did some magic tricks to get things on track. He told us that we would be put on the schedule for the following morning, and that the neurosurgeon in charge of my case would be Dr. Michael McDermott. We soon met with Dr. McDermott and immediately liked him. Besides having the Charlie Wilson stamp of approval, I discovered an added reason for feeling completely comfortable with Dr. McDermott—he was a first-generation Irishman!

When Todd had laughingly raised the point that he wasn't sure that McDermott was old enough to be doing surgery, Dr. Wilson told us that the new cutting-edge stuff like Gamma Knife surgery was best done by the "kids" who could do it better than he. And after meeting with Mike McDermott, we all had the feeling that we were dealing with the guy who could get the job done for me.

Late that afternoon, Todd and Ginny took us to a hotel before they headed back to San Diego. For a few minutes the four of us stood next to the car and held on to each other. We had made an abrupt change in our plans, and it had all happened very quickly, but I really believed that we had made the right decision. I knew that I was heading to Gamma Knife surgery the next day, and I know it might sound crazy, but I was pumped! Finally, I felt that we were moving forward. As Todd and Ginny quickly brushed aside tears and gave us their good wishes, I turned to Gerri and again said, "I'm ready. Let's do it!"

This was really a gut reaction on my part. It was a feeling I had—and Gerri shared—that we had found the right place.

It obviously wasn't the surroundings themselves that inspired confidence, and I knew we had met good, competent doctors at the other facilities we had visited. But UCSF just felt right. I think there are times when you have to go with your instincts. Do your homework (or get Gerri to do it for you), but there's going to come a time when you have to make a decision. I hope you'll get to a place where it feels right. If you get that feeling, trust it. Believe it. And go for it!

#19 Go for It When the Treatment Sounds Right

When your loved one comes to believe in a treatment or specific doctor or facility, overcome any concerns you may have and back up the patient 100 percent. You'll have helped gather information, and presented it along with your opinions and best advice, but the final decisions about who, what, where, and when really need to be made by the patient. Once those decisions have been made, it's time for the advocate to get on board and be fully enthusiastic about the patient's choice.

Gerri

"Sit down. Right now. Sit down in that chair."

The curt, crisp words came from Dr. McDermott. I'd just walked into the room after filling out some paperwork and Brian was in a chair facing me, a nurse behind him. As soon as I sat down, I understood why the doctor was concerned. He was literally using a screwdriver to drive a screw into my husband's forehead. The nurse stood behind Brian, trying to keep his head steady. They assured me they had applied local anesthetic, but while Brian didn't make a whimper, it was clear he was in great discomfort.

I couldn't do anything to help him, but I knew that one of the best things I could do was not let Brian know just how terrible the whole thing looked. It was awful. I couldn't reach out to touch him, so as I sat a few feet away, I hummed him a song. You have no way of knowing how terrible my voice is, and my humming isn't much better, but it was the only thing I could think of at the time. "The Minstrel Boy" is an Irish song about a boy going off to war and Brian had often told me it was his father's favorite. I have no idea what brought that particular tune to mind at the time, but given the circumstances, it was somehow appropriate.

When Dr. McDermott finished with the last of the four screws, they attached what resembled a weird metal halo onto Brian's head. Brian glanced up at me apprehensively.

"How do I look?"

"If you move your tongue back and forth and ask for fava beans, you'll be a dead ringer for Hannibal Lector."

Everyone laughed and the doctors led Brian off for a pre-surgery MRI. During the surgery itself, which took about an hour and a half, I sat in the waiting area visualizing what they were doing to him.

Although the surgery is called Gamma Knife, there really is no knife or scalpel involved. Brian's head was immobilized inside what looked like a gigantic football helmet. I knew that after being wheeled into a heavy steel cylinder, he would be receiving small doses of radiation, converging on the tumors from each of 201 different holes in the helmet. When these beams intersected at the site of the tumor, they delivered a highly concentrated dose of radiation. The beauty of this procedure was that the surrounding brain tissue only got a very weak dose of radiation, reducing radiation damage.

Brian would later wow people with his explanation of his brain tumors being "zapped" or "fried" by the Gamma Knife. The reality is far less romantic. The gamma rays don't really destroy the tumor, but instead they alter the DNA of the tumor itself so that it can no longer multiply. A tumor needs to keep growing or replicating itself in order to survive. But because the DNA has been altered, when the cells of the tumor try to grow, the tumor eventually dies off.

As we'd sat in our hotel room the night before, I had spoken with Brian in terms of his being the beneficiary of some type of Star Wars technology. However, the sight of Brian sitting next to an ordinary Sears Craftsman red toolbox, while the doctor used an actual screwdriver to fasten the halo onto Brian's head, gave me a big jolt of reality. Any thoughts I had of Star Wars were gone and I quickly came crashing back from outer space.

Brian

The Gamma Knife team consisted of the neurosurgeon, Dr. McDermott, and the physicist and the radiation oncologist, who together did the computations and the mapping of the gamma rays. I was completely awake during the procedure and in my typically weird way, was almost euphoric with the thought that the tumors inside my head were on their way to being destroyed. Facedown in my halo and strapped inside a large helmet full of holes for the gamma rays, I was maneuvered into a huge cylinder. The room I was in was lined with lead walls, and the doctors performed the procedure from another room, safe from radiation exposure. In this way, I was completely cut off from the outside world. Cut off, except for the microphone next to me. Obviously, my doctors had not been forewarned about my affinity for microphones!

At some point, I started doing something for which I've gained some renown. I began telling Irish stories, and eventually started to sing Irish songs. The team found this so amusing that they called in a doctor from another department in the hospital. He'd been born in Ireland and, amused by my buffoonery, began to sing along with me. Back and forth we sang Irish songs, and Star Wars technology gave way to "Galway Bay."

The procedure itself lasted only about an hour or so, and following that, I was taken to a room to recuperate for a few hours. I was given some medication to take care of some pain at the sites where the halo had been secured. I dozed a bit, waking intermittently to see Gerri in a chair by my bedside. When it was obvious that I had suffered no ill effects from the surgery, I was released.

It was pretty amazing. At two in the afternoon, I had undergone a procedure designed to eradicate two brain tumors. At seven that evening, I was ready to leave the hospital with no outward sign of what I had gone through. No outward sign other than two round, nickel-size Band-Aids located about two inches above and to the outside corner of each of my eyebrows. As Gerri and I waited for the elevator, a janitor came strolling up with a big bucket full of mops and brooms. The man looked at me, then at the elevator, then back to me again.

With a shy smile and a voice worthy of Morgan Freeman, he turned to me and said, "Looks like they done took your antlers off."

The next day, I had a follow-up with Dr. McDermott. He indicated that everything looked fine and pronounced me "good to go." Exactly the words I wanted to hear.

"Gerri and I are supposed to be in Dublin on June twentieth. Can I go?" I asked.

That first night back in May when we had gotten the diagnosis, one of the first calls we made was to the Parkers, the friends we were to meet up with in Italy. We called to tell them not to pick us up at the airport, that we'd had a change of plans. When they heard the excuse I had for canceling our trip, we had to do some fast talking to convince them to stay in Italy and enjoy themselves.

In my usual overoptimistic and sometimes unrealistic way, I promised them that Gerri and I would fly over and meet them in Dublin in a month. By then, I assured them, we would have everything under control. I had talked about this upcoming trip to Ireland many times in those first few miserable weeks of my diagnosis. For me, holding out the thought of this trip had helped pull me through some of my darker moments. I guess I'm a real believer in the carrot-versus-the-stick philosophy.

Set Short-Term Goals and Rewards

Advocate Tip
#20

When Brian was dealing with the terrible headaches caused by the brain tumors, I agreed with his idea that we would go to Ireland just as soon as we finished with the Gamma Knife. I am the first to admit that I really didn't think he would be physically able to go at that point, but I encouraged him to believe that he could. Later, when he was going through a vaccine program in Dallas, I planned our trips in such a way that we could go down to Puerto Vallarta, Mexico, for our annual vacation. Every year for the preceding ten years, we'd been able to join friends at the same place, same time, every year. Puerto Vallarta has served as an important goal for us, and getting there has served as an important marker of our success.

It's not just about the vacation itself and the rest and relaxation your body gets. Having a specific reward to look forward to can give your patient something positive to focus on and help carry him or her through the dark moments. Whether it's a vacation or the birth of a grandchild or attending an important reunion, having something specific to look forward to is so important for your patient. Give positive feedback, saying that he or she is going to be well enough to take part. Provide something to aim for when it's tough going. And then, make sure you get there!

Gerri had gone along with my plans to go to Ireland from day one. Later, I learned that she was just playing along with me, never dreaming that this would come true! In her effort to keep my spirits up, she had even booked our flights, all the while convinced that the doctors or my medical condition would prevent us from going.

Now Dr. McDermott laughed. He thought I was kidding. "Brian, you just had the Gamma Knife yesterday, and June twentieth is only ten days from now. Are you serious?"

"You bet. We've missed a month in Italy and I promised our friends we'd meet them in Ireland. Is there any medical reason I can't go?"

My neurosurgeon was dumbfounded. He thought about it and then replied, "Medically, I guess I don't see any reason why you can't go. I'm just a little surprised."

After some admonitions on taking care of myself and some definitive instructions to Gerri, he laughed and said, "Say hello to Ireland for me. Go have a good time."

I intended to. I was going to live my life as if I had cancer, but not as if it had me.

Chapter Five

PUSH THE ENVELOPE

Why not go out on a limb? That's where the fruit is.
—WILL ROGERS

Gerri

I can't describe the wonderful feelings we experienced after the Gamma Knife procedure. Finally, after weeks of tossing and turning every night, finally—finally—we had done something! We had taken the steps necessary to get rid of the first two things that could kill Brian, the brain tumors. We were almost giddy with relief.

Brian was still taking heavy doses of steroids, so Gamma Knife surgery or not, as soon as he was dismissed from the hospital, the first thing we did was find a restaurant. His need for food ruled. We called the kids and then with a few other key calls, got my new phone tree in action. Everyone was amazed. Few of them had known that we were heading to San Francisco, so the call saying that Brian had completed the Gamma Knife surgery and that we were making calls from a restaurant had our friends and family stunned. As everyone kept repeating, it was a medical miracle.

We were both very upbeat, very happy—and very exhausted. When they talk about how difficult things are for the person who has to sit and wait, they're not kidding. I had done "nothing" for twelve hours, but by the time I got Brian to bed that night, I felt as if I'd run a marathon.

The euphoria lasted longer for Brian than it did for me. He spent much of the next few days regaling everyone with stories about the procedure. I was already over that and back into my research mode. We might have "zapped" the immediate enemy, the brain tumors, but I could not forget that the underlying cause, the melanoma, still remained.

I spent those next couple of weeks doing more research and making more phone calls about the various melanoma treatment programs across the country. We were beginning to narrow our focus to those at UCSF and the John Wayne Cancer Center. Each had a different type of vaccine protocol, and Brian was considered a good candidate to go into the program at either institute. As one physician told him, "Except for the cancer, you're really healthy." That cancer, though, was obviously a problem, a dreaded, ugly monster that I knew was still on the attack, eating away at my husband.

Our schedule called for a follow-up MRI of the brain on July 9th up in San Francisco. In a month, we would find out if the Gamma Knife had been successful. In a month, we would find out if we'd been able to stop the growth of the two tumors inside Brian's brain. I couldn't decide if I wanted that month to crawl or fly by.

Make Use of a University-Affiliated Medical Center

If you are frozen by the diagnosis of cancer or any other disease or illness that life tosses at you, and you have no solid idea as to where to go for treatment, consider starting at a teaching institution—a medical center affiliated with a university. These places usually have teaching and research facilities, which may give you your best shot at both cutting-edge technology and research. And if the teaching institution in your area doesn't, ask for input from them as to where you should go. A good question to start with is: "If your wife or mother (or husband or father) had this diagnosis, where would *you* take her?" That question should give you some answers to get started with your search.

Teaching facilities often attract dedicated, intelligent doctors with a passion for understanding and curing disease. If you don't have a good starting point for getting the best treatment, think about going to a teaching medical center.

Summer had begun, and in addition to figuring out how to attack Brian's melanoma, we tried to get on with the business of living. We went to baseball games and lunch with friends. Brian went to the office and continued to work on making the changes to his business that needed to be made. The kids visited frequently. In short, we were doing our best to live life to the fullest.

There were plenty of medical appointments during that time, too. Brian was having blood work, and suffering blinding headaches as a result of having to come off steroids to be eligible for the clinical trials we were pursuing. I was learning a tremendous amount about my new role as advocate. As we went in and out of doctors' offices, I was getting plenty of practice in remaining vigilant as we pursued our various options.

Brian

Remember, I am an experienced trial lawyer of thirty years. I have represented doctors and have also brought suits against doctors, and I believe that although the world is full of fine doctors, it's absolutely true that you have to be very, very careful. With the emergence of managed care, HMOs, and the ever-present bottom-line mentality forced on the medical world by insurance companies, doctors are often overworked and end up having to rush from one patient to another. I may have been a tiger in the courtroom, but as a patient I found that when I was in pain, or what I came to think of as a fog caused by that pain, I developed a strong tendency to accept, accept, accept. I know the statistics on preventable medical deaths. Trust me on this: an advocate who is intelligent, and assertive, and willing to ask questions can improve your chances of survival.

Find Your Own Voice as an Advocate

Young attorneys could often be found sitting in the front rows of the courtroom during Brian's trials hoping to learn something. At the end of the trial, they often approached him, asking for advice on how to be successful. Brian's standard reply was, "Be yourself." Those same words are good advice for someone now in the role of an advocate. Be yourself.

I'm the first to admit that I'm not the shy, retiring type. My style of advocacy is much more "in your face" than it probably should be, and when things aren't going well, I don't back off. For example, if someone told me that they could not admit Brian to the hospital when he needed immediate care, I had no problem going into what Brian calls my "don't mess with Gerri" voice and insisting that I get to see the head of nursing or admissions, or the head of the hospital. Early on in this battle, I decided that I wasn't in this to win the Miss Congeniality award. I was in this to get the best possible care for my husband and I didn't care what they said about me behind my back.

This doesn't mean that my style will work for you. I think that using a softer, more gentle approach can also be helpful when you're advocating on behalf of your patient. And if you're a person who breaks down in tears when things are going poorly? I've seen that style work wonders, too.

Whatever your personality is, whatever your style, however you deal with authority or critical situations, the important thing to remember is that you are an advocate. The style isn't as important as the fact that you're willing to be there, asking questions and when necessary standing up to the "white coats" on behalf of your patient.

You can be polite and soft-spoken or brassy and bold, but never lose sight of your goal. If your patient is not getting the care he or she needs, do not hesitate to step in. So be yourself. But above all, be an advocate.

Brian

One night just before our trip to Ireland, I was feeling better than usual and able to think more clearly. Enjoying a warm Southern California evening, Gerri and I sat out on our patio. During the past few days, we had spent lots of time and energy going from doctor to doctor and city to city and by now, we had witnessed some pretty gut-wrenching things. Seeing my own brain tumors on an MRI screen was an eye-opener, but seeing the effects of cancer on real people was something else. All those cancer victims, walking around the hallways of hospitals, pushing their IV poles. What I found so disturbing was that their eyes seemed vacant. To me, it looked as if many of them had given up hope. I don't know if the people I saw were all just having really bad days, but they didn't seem to be walking around with the sense that they were getting anywhere at all. Hell, I could push a pole around the world if I had to, but I'd need to have a sense that doing it was going to help achieve something. Like living. Not just being alive. Living.

That night out on the patio, Gerri and I talked about the fact that we didn't want to forego quality of life for quantity of life. I had watched my mother suffer for several years from multiple myeloma, a cancer of the bones. She had put up a great battle, and I was enormously proud of her, but in the end she lost the fight. And the end had been miserable. And after watching my brother's decline, I had also talked with Gerri about not wanting to live in a condition where I was severely mentally impaired. Now I asked her to make sure that if I ever got to that stage where there was no hope left, she would let me stop fighting and just live out the rest of my days as best I could.

She nodded her understanding.

Know Your Patient's Wishes

Advocate Tip
#23

It may seem obvious, but as early on in your patient's illness as you can, I encourage you to have this difficult conversation. What extraordinary measures, if any, does your patient want taken to prolong life? Does he want to be on a respirator? When, if ever, does she want the "plug pulled"?

Encourage your patient to have a living will and a power of attorney for health care purposes. While the titles may vary from state to state, essentially these are documents in which the patient decides at what point he no longer wishes to have extraordinary methods used to keep him alive. This is a highly individual and personal decision and there is no one answer that will fit everyone.

In recent years, I've found that every time we check into a hospital, they ask, "Do you have a living will and a power of attorney for health care? If so, can we have it so we can make a copy of it for your file? If not, would you like to look at a standardized form that we have, and use it to make those decisions for yourself?" This whole subject can make anyone squeamish and uncomfortable, but if it is presented to patients in the light of their being able to help control decisions for themselves, it can help give them comfort and peace of mind.

Clearly my fight was just beginning, and having this conversation with my wife didn't mean I had any intention of giving up. Gerri's research and the information she had made her realize that we didn't have much to lose by being aggressive. That night, she again talked about the need for us to push the envelope. She made it seem like the smart, intelligent, progressive, and aggressive thing to do. That attitude of going on the attack, not sitting back and being passive, was one that resonated with me. Gerri knew that she would have a willing partner in me to go outside the box in our battle against cancer.

Advocate Tip
#24

Push the Envelope

It is worth taking a look at the concept of "pushing the envelope," a phrase I think was used by Chuck Yeager and other test pilots when they were pushing all limitations on both man and their airplanes by going fast enough to break the sound barrier. Brian has been a risk taker for much of his life, and although I don't put myself in his category, when I look back I realize that during my lifetime, I've taken more than a few risks myself. So our personalities certainly predisposed us to the concept of pushing the envelope. That, plus the cold realization that we simply weren't presented with any really viable alternatives. I think that if we had seen a good track record for more traditional methods in the treatment of Brian's cancer, we may well have gone that route—but it's a lot easier to take risks when all your other options look like dead ends. In too many ways, we simply had nothing to lose.

Early on in our battle, I learned that no one oncologist can know all there is to know about any particular type of cancer. That holds true for any type of medical specialist and any type of medical problem. There is just too much information out there, too much new research being done, too many new clinical trials going on, to keep up with all of it. There may be something new, something that hasn't created much of a stir yet in the traditional medical world, or hasn't made it into the medical journals. That something might be the one thing that will work for your patient. As the advocate, you're in a perfect position to help push the envelope. You need to take a look at all the newer options while at the same time considering the more traditional approaches. That means exploring clinical trials.

I know the concept of trying something unproven, a treatment that has little, if any, track record, can be frightening. But especially if your options are limited, it really is something you should consider. We're not advocating going to a foreign country to swallow almond pits. We're talking about staying within the medical world as you know it, yet taking a look at the very newest thinking that's taking place.

Many university medical schools are working on clinical trials involving all aspects of medicine, not just cancer. Call them or go on their websites and find out if they're doing something that might be of help. Even if you aren't in the position to travel around the country in your search for a treatment, you just might discover that there's something new being done in your own backyard. Remember, the life of someone you love is at stake. There's simply no good reason to not do some research and then discuss the information you've collected with your doctor. You may find something that resonates with you, something you can use to push the envelope. To paraphrase Robert Kennedy, who paraphrased the Jewish scholar Hillel, "If not you, who? If not now . . . when?"

See page 211 for resources to help you explore clinical trials.

Brian

June 20th came, the day of our much-anticipated trip to Ireland. Along with the Parkers, we met up with some other fellow San Diegans and Sherry Bahrambeygui and her soon-to-be fiancé,

Pat Hosey. It was a great trip, made even better because I'd just come through the Gamma Knife.

I was on a roll the entire three days in Ireland. The doctors had put me on a decreasing amount of steroids in the hope of weaning me off them, but I was still under their effect. My face was so blown up it looked like a full moon. But more significantly, I now had incredible energy and was on some kind of crazy sleep schedule. What little sleep I was able to get seemed to be during the day. At night I could go forever! Gerri said I was like the worst infant in the world. At two in the morning, long after the pubs had closed, I still wanted to party, sing, and laugh.

In an effort to allow Gerri to get some much needed sleep, friends took turns spending time with me in the wee hours of the morning when I was still raring to go. One evening I spent time telling John Clark, a friend from San Diego, about the Gamma Knife procedure. But unlike the others who had merely listened politely to my story, John was really fascinated by it. He did some research into the latest Gamma Knife technology and soon discovered what he considered to be a better mousetrap. An explanation of this newer Rotating Gamma Knife system can be found on page 214, and while I don't pretend to have any knowledge of cutting-edge scientific technology, I like the idea that my procedure may have given rise to John's vision of pushing the envelope in this field.

One of the highlights of our trip was the engagement of Sherry and Pat, which they announced at a black-tie dinner held in the magical setting of Powers Court, a castle just south of Dublin. The guests rose to toast the couple and it was one of those moments when all the planets were aligned. The setting was startlingly beautiful, I had decided that the Gamma Knife had been successful, I'd just experienced an emotional reunion with the Parkers and our other friends, and I was surrounded by people who all joined in wishing me well. I stood with my arms wrapped around Gerri. The video made that evening shows an exceptionally happy moon-faced man. It was an evening I'll never forget.

Gerri

The video does tell the story. Brian was ebullient; his joy of life never leaves his face. And next to him? One exhausted lady with an ever watchful eye constantly trained on her husband. At times it was difficult for me to listen to Brian as he regaled our friends with the story of how the Gamma Knife had "taken care of" the brain tumors. As far as he was concerned, those tumors were gone. I wasn't going to rain on Brian's parade, but I was more cautious in my optimism.

I saw this trip as a respite for Brian from what we were about to face. There were the cancerous lymph nodes we knew would have to be removed. In addition, the doctors in San Francisco had taken me aside to share their fear that the presence of more than one brain tumor indicated that the cancer had already "seeded." The doctors told me they felt pretty certain that Brian's next MRI would show numerous small tumors scattered throughout his brain. I hadn't told this to Brian or anyone other than the children, and now, Susan Parker. I wanted to have him soak up every minute of happiness that he could in Ireland. While everyone thought that I was simply worn out trying to keep up with the "Energizer Bunny on steroids," I think I was more exhausted by trying to fake a good time. I was all too aware that Brian's fun would probably be fleeting. So while Brian was singing "Galway Bay," my mind was focused on more practical problems. I was saying prayers that he would live long enough to be with us for Christmas, six months away. I was wishing with every ounce of strength I had that I could *make* that happen, even as I knew I couldn't.

Don't Try to Control Everything

You can't control everything, so just do the best you can. Sounds simple, right? Actually, I think it's one of the most difficult things you will do as an advocate. Whatever crisis you're dealing with, be it cancer or a heart condition or a brain injury, one of the biggest lessons you have to learn is that you can only do so much. There are things beyond your control and you must accept that. Ten years later, I have to admit this is still one of life's lessons that doesn't come easily to me.

I did have a role model in learning to relinquish control. For years, I had watched Brian fighting for his clients. He was always convinced that he would win their case, but that didn't always happen—it's just not possible. As an advocate I had to remind myself, over and over again, that I could do my very best, try my hardest, and still not be able to guarantee a good outcome. In my mind it was my job to save his life, but I might do my very best and still he might die.

Too many advocates know this. The best advocate we know, Russ Block, broke all the standards in the care he gave his wife, Judy Keep. Judy, the first woman appointed to the Federal Court in San Diego, and Russ, an attorney and longtime law professor, fought a ferocious battle with Judy's ovarian cancer for three years. We watched with heartache as they lost that fight on September 14, 2004. But it wasn't for lack of trying. I don't think it's possible for anyone to surpass the kind of loving care and comfort that Russ bestowed on Judy. His dedication, and the valiant fight that she put up, kept her alive far longer than anyone thought possible, and of equal importance, kept her as comfortable and pain-free as possible. That's saying a lot.

During these past ten years, Brian and I have seen better advocates than I watch helplessly as their loved ones lost the battle. Did they fail in their role as an advocate? From the depths of my being, I can say, "Absolutely not."

As advocates, they had the courage to be there. They had the courage to face up to the white coats. They had the courage to ask the needed questions. They had the strength to sit in the waiting rooms, or by the bedside, always ready to help. They had stepped outside themselves and done things they never thought they could do. They became advocates and simply by assuming that role, they had succeeded. You can make a huge contribution in this battle simply by accepting your role as advocate, but be gentle with yourself. No matter how hard you try, you can't control everything.

One month after the Gamma Knife, we were back in San Francisco. As we sat in the UCSF Medical Center hallway, waiting for the results of Brian's latest MRI, I felt nauseated. Since we'd come back from Ireland, I had tried to prepare Brian for the possibility that there might be more brain tumors without letting him know that the doctors thought this was a probability.

When Dr. Wara, the radiation oncologist, came through the door with a huge grin on his face, I wanted to hug him. So I did. There in the hallway, the doctor told us that the MRI looked great. The smaller tumor in the occipital lobe appeared to be about the same size as before, but they expected it to decrease in size. The large tumor over the left temporal lobe showed the center of the tumor to be collapsing and the ring of the tumor diminishing in size. And not only that: there were no new tumors! None.

Dr. Wara shook his head in wonder and delight. This was good news beyond all expectation. We have learned along the way that the doctors truly appreciate being able to give, and share in, good news. For oncologists and neurosurgeons, it doesn't happen often enough.

When we met with Dr. McDermott, he was equally pleased but said that although the swelling caused by the tumors had diminished, he wanted Brian to continue on the steroids for an additional six weeks. This caused me concern, as I knew that more steroids would continue to suppress Brian's immune system. Not only that, but all the research I had done indicated that Brian couldn't get into any of the vaccine programs until he was off steroids—which meant we couldn't begin to deal with the underlying cause of the tumors, the cancer itself. So while the news on the brain tumors was great, I began to shift my focus to other areas. Now we had to deal with the tumor in his lymph nodes and start fighting on the second front of our war. The battle against melanoma was just beginning.

Brian

I didn't understand at that point Gerri's concerns about more brain tumors. I was focused on the two I had, and the thought that we had dealt with those. I was happy to have my optimistic outlook confirmed by the MRI, which showed them to be collapsing. Again, I had a mental image, this time of tumors imploding inside my head. Totally inaccurate, but a great image for me to focus on.

While we were up in San Francisco, we met with the melanoma specialists at UCSF and discussed their vaccine programs. The doctors had an upbeat outlook on the success rate of their vaccine—and although a success rate of 20 percent might not sound great to some, I absolutely believed that I would be in the 20 percent grouping.

Gerri and I both liked the idea of a vaccine, or some type of therapy along those lines, rather than a more traditional chemo approach. Maybe it was because we had been raised during the successful implementation of the Salk vaccine against polio. To us, a vaccine or anything else used to boost or enhance the immune system seemed like a positive approach. And since there were very few Stage IV melanoma survivors around who could advocate on behalf of chemotherapy, that approach—at least for my problem—continued to sound old-fashioned and negative to us. In our continuing saga, the doctors sent us back home with the understanding that I would have to be back at UCSF in late July for the surgery necessary to remove my cancerous lymph nodes. After that, we hoped to get on with the fight against those ugly little SOBs racing through my blood.

Gerri

In retrospect, having Brian remain on steroids longer than we had anticipated gave us some breathing room to better make our decision on a choice of a treatment program. I kept in touch with the various programs with updates on Brian's medical progress. And they all kept calling us. It seemed everyone wanted Brian to be in their program. Obviously, each entity truly thought that they had the best available option for Brian, and in addition, Brian was a great candidate for each program. Except for Stage IV melanoma, he was in great health, he had a great attitude, and he wasn't afraid of stepping outside the box. In fact, he relished it.

The last half of July was another one of those difficult times for me as we weighed one vaccine program against another. Again I had that feeling of being whipsawed back and forth while trying to make the best decision possible. When we listened to the merits of each program, we would get excited as it sounded like that was the one we should choose. But then the next one came along, and we would lean toward that one.

It was hard to make the decision based on medical information alone. By their very nature, these programs were all highly experimental and they didn't have much of a track record to mark their success. In most instances, it was just too early to know if any of them would really work. I began to narrow our choices down to a program that would keep us essentially at home. Although I had no problem with traveling for a few days or weeks in order to get Brian the best treatment, I believed that he would fare better if he was able to be around the people he loved, able to tap into the incredible support network we had. While I said that we would go anywhere, we were in effect limiting ourselves to Los Angeles or San Francisco unless something else came along to knock our socks off.

And it did.

Brian

Toward the end of July, we experienced one of those moments when you get to believe that some of the good you've done in the past has come full circle. Several years before, I had been contacted by Dr. Maurizio Zanetti, who asked me to represent him in a lawsuit. Although I couldn't take his case, I sent him to a friend and great attorney and I followed the case to see how it was proceeding. A cancer research doctor at the University of California, San Diego, Dr. Zanetti specialized in the field of immunotherapy and at the time of my diagnosis was working on a type of vaccine therapy of his own. This research was still in the very early conceptual stage, and certainly not something that would be available for me. When he heard about my illness, though, Dr. Zanetti reached out his hand and offered to help in any way he could.

Gerri told him that the research she had done into standard treatment didn't show much promise and had led us to the point of wanting to push the envelope and get into a clinical trial program. Dr. Zanetti told us that he would began mining his contacts throughout the medical world, both in the USA and abroad, to determine what effective therapy was available that might be of help to me. What he learned didn't give him much optimism. But he continued his search for something that might work.

A week or so after he first met with us, Maurizio came to our home with news that he had determined that the best option for me was something called dendritic-cell vaccine therapy, which had been done in Germany and Switzerland. Although it was in its very early stages, the results had been very good and the therapy showed great promise. He told us that in his opinion, the other therapies we were considering would not prove to be effective. He said that he agreed with our idea of pushing the envelope but thought that the vaccines we were considering were too "old" to push any envelopes. What he didn't tell us was that he had been told by many physicians and other researchers that the only thing I was going to be pushing would be daisies!

Within a day or so, Maurizio gave us further information that was of even greater interest. He told us that he had heard through the medical grapevine that a former colleague of his from Paris, Dr. Jacques Banchereau, had been recruited by a medical facility in Texas to begin work on a dendritic-cell vaccine program there. He had no more information than that, but Maurizio ended the conversation in his classic Italian accent with the words, "I will find him for you." *

*For Dr. Maurizio Zanetti's insights regarding hope and not giving up too soon, see page 207.

About two weeks later, Dr. Zanetti called with wonderful news. He had located his former colleague, who had just been appointed the lead research scientist for a new melanoma vaccine program at the Baylor Institute of Immunology in Dallas. They had spoken by phone and discussed the possibility of my enrolling as a patient in their clinical trial. In one of those incredibly lucky circumstances I seem to be drawn to, the chief medical officer of the program, Dr. Joseph Fay, just "happened" to be vacationing in the San Diego area. After a few urgent phone calls tracking him down, we learned that he would be happy to meet with us the next morning, just before he was due to return to Dallas. As Gerri said, the stars were in alignment once again.

When we talked to Dr. Fay and later with Dr. Banchereau, I learned that if all my tests met their criteria, I would be enrolled as their first patient. The idea of being the initial guinea pig didn't scare me off at all, but now Gerri seemed to want me to wait and perhaps be the second guinea pig. It will come as no surprise to you by now that I actually relished the thought of being first! I had been taking chances since I was a kid, and it was no time to stop now. That attitude had brought me great rewards in my life, and I believed that it would work for me now. I was really charged up with the prospect of this new vaccine therapy.

Gerri

This was a classic case of "be careful what you wish for." Brian was excited about getting into the program at Baylor. Me, not so much. Since the day we received the diagnosis, I had been selling Brian on the idea that we'd be like the guys on *Star Trek* and "go where no man has gone before"; still I didn't feel ready for him to be the *first* patient for this program. Second, third, or fourth sounded a lot better. But Brian had come to believe deeply in the program at Baylor, and I recognized how important that belief was. And the more I learned about the dendritic-cell vaccine, the more I became a believer, too.

Dr. Banchereau, the director of the Baylor Institute for Immunology Research in Dallas, described dendritic cells as the generals of the immune-system army. I learned from my research that dendritic cells are shaped like spiny starfish and roam the body, hunting for pathogens that cause disease. When they find something, they carry it to a lymph node, where they "recruit and train" T-cells to recognize and fight the invaders. Scientists are discovering more and more about the important role dendritic cells play in our immune system's response to illness. And biotechnology companies are developing new vaccines all the time. Some of these consist of dendritic cells loaded with bits of patients' own tumors, and are intended to activate the immune system against a patient's particular form of cancer. More information on dendritic cells and how they work can be found on page 214.

It's a very complex technology and it wasn't easy to boil this all down into a concept that we could understand, relate to, and want to rally around. I spent quite a bit of time trying to get a handle on it all. In addition to doing a lot of reading, I again asked a lot of questions.

Advocate Tip
#26 Make Doctors Speak in Language You Understand

One of the most important questions you can ask as an advocate is: "Doctor, could you please explain that to me in English so that I can understand what you're saying?"

Every profession has its own jargon, and with its vocabulary based on Latin and Greek, that's especially true of the medical profession. While most of us have no problem asking the guy selling us a sound system to explain the difference between a woofer and a tweeter, for some inexplicable reason we are afraid to question a doctor. Don't be. As the advocate, one of your main goals is to listen and learn what is being done, or can be done, for your patient. It's simply impossible to do that if the words you are hearing are incomprehensible to you. Unless you are among the small group who learned Latin in school, medical jargon is a language you will not understand. You will do your patient no good at all if you simply sit back and nod while understanding very little of what is being said.

Here's another instance of how useful keeping a journal will be. "Doctor speak" is not only incomprehensible, it is often spoken at warp speed. But as long as you take notes, you can later look up the terminology, or discuss recommendations with other people, and then contact the physician with questions or concerns.

I know it can be intimidating, but it's absolutely vital that you speak up. Even medical professionals want advocates by their sides when they are patients. So ask questions; ask for explanations in terms *you* understand. Ask over and over again, until you *do* understand it. Yes,

it is more than likely that the doctor or nurse is in a hurry, but don't be intimidated into shutting up! Your patient's life is at stake, and you are the one helping to determine the course of action needed.

Brian had gone through the Gamma Knife, and we counted on that to take care of the brain tumors. Now we decided that a dendritic-cell vaccine was the route to follow in order to deal with the systemic cancer itself. With little else on the horizon, we placed all our hopes in this basket.

The only catch was that while we were ready, they weren't. The Baylor team was waiting to receive FDA approval to start the program, and they thought it would come any day now. Brian and I talked about it ourselves and then with our closest circle of family and friends. In the end, we decided that this was worth waiting for. It was a huge decision to wait to be the first guinea pig, and one I, if not Brian, lost a lot of sleep over.

It was essential that we get our minds off all that could go wrong. To this end, we turned our focus to home and family.

Chapter Six

TAKE CARE OF
THE HOME FRONT

Death is more universal than life;
everyone dies but not everyone lives.

—A. SACHS

Gerri

"Everybody look this way. On the count of three—one, two,
three. Cheese."

Perched on a rock outcropping along a stretch of beach in
San Diego, the combined family of Brian and Gerri Monaghan
squinted into the late afternoon sun. Anyone walking by would
probably have assumed that they were witnessing a simple
family photo, or even an early sitting for a Christmas card. It all
looked so perfect. But just as with most of the family photos you
receive at Christmastime, there was a story that didn't show in
any of our faces. Brian's cancer was undetectable on the surface,
but none of us forgot for a second that it was there.

We had gathered all the kids and their spouses together in San
Diego. I hired a photographer to take a family picture and then
we all headed back to the house. A day or so before this, I told
Brian some story about always having wanted a video camera,
and I think he was still deep enough in that foggy stage that
he went along with the idea. He probably understood exactly

what I was trying to do. In any event, I bought the video camera and we began using it. We used it extensively over the next few days. Everyone was trying hard not to make it sound as if they were recording some last statements at the request of the prison warden, and Brian did his best to make it all fun.

Brian had always wanted to integrate our two families into one, and this crisis was a good catalyst for accomplishing that. All four of our "kids" were grown and living in three different cities at the time of our marriage, so it hadn't been easy to cement a family bond, but now Brian felt a more urgent need to make that happen. Of even greater importance to him was his desire to bring his children, Kathi and Patrick, closer together as brother and sister. No matter how optimistic he was, we were all facing the realization that none of us would be around forever. Brian really wanted to make another effort at family unity.

Brian

The evening we all gathered together at our home was beautiful and moonlit with everybody trying their best to be optimistic. We kept it as light as possible, but there was no denying that concern, even fear, was an undercurrent. I've come to understand that we all react in different ways to a crisis situation, and our family was no different. It seemed to me that Gerri's children and their spouses had a good grasp on the uphill battle I was facing. I think it was much more difficult for my own children to deal with that reality. When they were young they had watched my mother, who lived with us, suffer greatly before her death from cancer. Now, it seemed difficult for them to have to think in terms of that same ending for me. Over the next few weeks, I made sure that I spent time reassuring them that I wasn't ready to pack it in yet. They had seen me overcome seemingly insurmountable odds in the past, and we all focused on my doing that now.

It's important for you as a patient to understand that your family members may well be having their own difficulties when it comes to dealing with your illness. Give them a break. Back away from any frustration you may have in this regard, and focus your energy on the fight at hand. Easier said than done, I know. But I believe that at this critical point in your life, you as a patient will need to put yourself and your own needs above the needs of others. I know that it's a thought contrary to what we usually believe, but it's vital at this moment in time. It will take every ounce of your strength, every bit of energy you have to focus on survival. If that means you have to put the needs of others on the back burner for a while, do it. You can refocus on others when you're feeling better, but you won't be able to help them at all if you are not around. This is a time in your life when you must be selfish. You must take care of yourself and gather all of your strength for what's ahead. Hopefully, you'll be able to take up the battles for others at another time.*

*For Kathi Vaughn's perspective on supporting a positive attitude, see page 208.

Gerri

The period after the Gamma Knife, when we were looking into vaccine options, was anything but uneventful. As is true for most families dealing with serious illness, life went on. The procedures and doctors' appointments took vast amounts of time and energy, but we were also dealing with major upheavals at Brian's office. And while our primary focus was on saving his life, we were also determined to live life to the fullest with whatever time we had. I didn't want to look back with any regrets. I wanted to be able to say we'd given it our all and enjoyed ourselves every step of the way. This meant some sorting of priorities.

Brian

By August of 1998, it became clear that I would have to take steps to deal with my law firm. What had been my life's blood, and in so many ways the focus of my life, had begun to get complicated even before my medical problems. Now the fault lines were magnified, as fear took hold and everyone's need to take care of his or her own future became paramount.

I started my law firm in 1975 and it had continued with a varying cast of characters and a damned good success rate for twenty-three years. But within a few months of my cancer diagnosis, the firm, which had often been described as a wheel with me as the center, began to disintegrate. To be honest, part of that was my fault: I loved trial work too much to watch the other lawyers in the firm step up and assume the mantle. I wasn't ready to let go.

Taking on major trials is like high-stakes poker. There were several years when I owed more than a million dollars on an individual case, and had my home and everything I owned on the line in the hope that we would prevail. But as I said, our success rate had been good, and we had done well.

When cancer struck, many reached the "obvious" conclusion that I would not survive more than a few months. Many of our clients panicked, believing that the guy they had chosen as their savior was abandoning them. As a result, the pressure on my partners and staff was enormous. Fear lurked in the hallways. Some people bailed almost immediately. Some, like Sherry Bahrambeygui, acted as I had hoped (she worked from home when she was pregnant and on prescribed bed rest). Mike Conger, too, stepped up and assumed enormous responsibility for the big case we had that remained on appeal. But I wasn't taking on new cases, and the firm was barely lurching along.

Some of these people had been with me for five, ten, fifteen years, and we had been through marriages, births, deaths, major successes, and heartbreaking defeats. We had worked long hours together down in the trenches, truly believing that we were making a difference in the lives of our clients, and had forged an incredible bond. When it became clear that Brian Monaghan, plaintiffs' lawyer, would not be back, it was time to shut it all down. We went through some painful negotiations, parceling out the remaining cases, but within a year or so of my cancer diagnosis it was basically over. The firm I had put so much into was gone.

It wasn't easy. No, that's not true—it was the pits. We all define ourselves in certain ways, and I had always seen myself as a trial lawyer. If you've spent your life building a meaningful career, I know you understand. To have your identity taken away from you in a major life-changing event isn't easy for anyone and it wasn't for me. But I simply didn't have the luxury of mooning over anything. I didn't have the luxury of allowing myself to be consumed by anger. I had to marshal all my strength and energy for a fight that had become far more important than any of my past legal battles.

In late July, momentarily leaving behind all the upheaval at my office, Gerri and I were back in San Francisco, this time to have a lymphadenectomy in which the cancerous lymph nodes were removed from my right axilla (that's medical terminology for armpit). First I had another round of CT scans and received great news. They didn't show any new signs of cancer. A day or so before this, Gerri and I had something else to celebrate: finally, after being on steroids for about two months, I was able to come off them. We both saw this as a major achievement. Maybe now I could start acting and feeling normal (or whatever my version of normal is). The lymph node surgery was easy to handle. I had it performed as an outpatient—I'm sure that they'll be doing drive-by heart surgery before too long!—and after checking in at nine in the morning, I was out of there by five.

Since I had sailed through the surgery, I thought the recovery would be easy. Wrong again. The week or so following this particular surgery was one of the more miserable times I had during my illness. First of all, they had inserted a drain in my armpit and told me that until the drain was removed, I had to take sponge baths. Well, I love my showers and this was like telling a fish to stay out of water. Gerri tried to help me with the sponge bath routine for several days, but she soon got sick of my whining and figured out a way to seal that area off with some combination of plastic wrap and tape. It was back to the showers for me.

Beyond this minor inconvenience, the next ten days were no picnic. The area around the drain became infected. But the toughest part was coming down off the steroids. The doctors had agreed to our request—born out of a desire to qualify for vaccine trials—for a much faster weaning process than usually recommended, and I paid a price for that. For about two weeks I was one miserable puppy. The wicked headaches I'd suffered before going on the steroids now returned. I had blurry vision and no appetite at all, and was totally lethargic all day but unable to sleep at night. Plus I was having meetings with my fellow attorneys at home.

The only good thing to come out of all this was that it gave me a sense of appreciation for what other cancer patients and people recovering from major surgery often have to go through. I admire people who stick through miserable times after chemo or an operation; they deserve tremendous credit for their strength and courage. I felt like a total wimp in comparison. My few weeks of "walking in their shoes" made me realize that anyone who goes through these kinds of physical ordeals for longer than I did is a hero in my book.

Taking it one step and then one day at a time, I got through it, mainly by hanging on to the hope of this new dendritic-cell vaccine program and doing what I could to keep my body strong.

Be Open to Complementary Alternative Medicine (CAM)

When we awoke on the morning of the diagnosis, neither Brian nor I was taking vitamins or supplements of any kind. One of the first things I read about cancer was that most researchers regarded it as a breakdown of the immune system. I decided that we needed to do everything we could to boost Brian's immune system, and vitamins seemed to be a logical extension of that.

We turned to a good friend, a chiropractor who was really into physical fitness and nutrition, Dr. Mark Cincotta. In fact, at that time Mark was serving as a team physician for an off-road bicycling team. Mark sat with me and wrote down a list of vitamins and supplements that he recommended for Brian.

Most of them can be generally categorized as antioxidants. Many medical people scoff at the world of vitamins, but unless someone can tell me that something is doing some harm, I'm open to what may be a potent ally. I know there are times when it seems as if you are getting conflicting information on whether or not some vitamin or supplement does or doesn't have value. I think you just have to go with the flow and try something until such time as it is proven ineffective. For example, researchers at San Diego's Moores Cancer Center have recently advocated taking 1,000 IU of vitamin D_3 as a way of reducing the risk of several types of cancer. I realize it's possible that within a few years, these same researchers may decide vitamin D doesn't help at all. But unless your doctor tells you that taking it will harm you in some way, why not give it a try?

While we were waiting for the vaccine program to get underway, there was almost nothing medically that we could do for Brian. With a strong belief in the ability of the mind to overcome so many things, I put a basket filled with these vitamins right on our kitchen counter and began a ritual of having Brian take them every morning. Whenever he forgot to take his pills I reminded him of how important they were in this battle. Since there was nothing else we could do for him, taking the vitamins and other supplements at least gave us a feeling of empowerment. It allowed both of us the desperately needed belief that we were doing *something*. That basket still sits in the same spot, and Brian takes the supplements to this day. We see no reason to stop.

We also looked at other avenues of complementary or alternative treatment. When Brian's headaches were at their worst, and he wasn't allowed to take much in the way of pain medication, he was open to trying something different—acupuncture. Although he didn't find this to have a long-lasting effect, the acupuncture treatments did provide him some relief. Tai chi, yoga, meditation, and massage are among the possible approaches you can try.

I think you should clear any of these "alternative" regimens with your physician before you start, to make certain that nothing interferes with your treatment plan, but beyond that, go for it. I take that back—we're not talking about going to Mexico for laetrile. We're talking about alternative treatments that are still within the confines of conventional medicine. See page 212 for a reliable resource on Complementary Alternative Medicine for cancer patients.

Gerri

"Ger, are you trying to get me ready for the funeral home?" Following Brian's gaze around our house, I began to see his point. I had bouquets of flowers tucked everywhere. Not only that, I had soothing music constantly playing in the background while lavender-scented candles burned, even in bright daylight. He was right. I guess I had taken my first attempts at trying to create a healing, stress-free environment for him a little too far.

The flowers and candles were just part of the story. I was also doing my best to keep things as quiet as possible. Brian's ability to sleep was so impaired by those early-stage headaches that we both cherished any sleep he could get. So every night before we went to bed I would take my clothes out for the next day, and a small bag filled with toothbrush and toiletries, and put them in the powder room so I could get dressed without bothering him. I carried the phone with me everywhere, even the bathroom, because it seemed that the return calls from the doctors always came when Brian had just fallen asleep.

Still, Brian seemed to wake up as soon as I made any movement in the bed. So every morning I did my version of the Pink Panther. Not that I would accuse my husband of snoring, but he does. On every exhale I'd make a slight movement, in hopes that any sound I made would be masked by his blubbering snore. First move the blanket. Next slide one foot over. Now the other. Put one foot on the floor. Now the other. Then tiptoe out. Ten years ago, we did not have one of those mattresses that allows one person to move without disturbing the other. We have one now. It sounds like a silly thing to recommend to you as an advocate, but if you can afford to buy one, do it. Sleep is critical.

The most all-encompassing, stress-reducing thing I did for Brian was to take over as many things as I could for him. By now, besides taking over as the firm's at-home office manager, I was handling and fielding all calls from doctors, hospitals, and clinics. I was also doing research. While not every patient wants to turn over ancillary duties, Brian did. This allowed me to handle most of the bad news and filter any of the information I gave to him. It's not a plan that would work for everyone but it was working for us, allowing Brian to concentrate on staying optimistic and looking forward with hope—not fear and despair.

In short, we established a new division of duties. Brian says he took responsibility for the weather and I was in charge of everything else. As long as we stayed in sunny San Diego, he did well! I think it was during this time frame that I came up with the saying, "My Husband, the Princess." As always, as best we could, we've maintained our sense of humor. You just do what you need to do to keep going forward. And if you can treat your patient like royalty, do it.

Advocate Tip #28 | Create a Stress-Free Environment

Studies have shown that stress exacerbates symptoms of disease across the board. So make a list of all the things, from handling calls to safeguarding sleep, that you can do to create a relaxing environment for your patient. Then implement them. No matter how goofy you might feel at first, your patient will appreciate your efforts.

Brian

While we were in the process of getting into a vaccine program, Gerri and I began to focus on the other important issues of our life. The fundamental reality is that life has changed for you and everyone around you. You're walking a tightrope. In order to give yourself the best shot at a successful outcome, you have to convince yourself that you are going to survive. Yet at the very same time, you have to be able to step back and realize that you must help yourself and your family prepare for the possibility of your death. No matter how much or how little time you'll have in fighting a disease, you have been given the gift of enough time. This is one of the areas where I think cancer, or any other life-threatening illness, can be a gift. Unlike that car accident or fatal heart attack, a protracted illness can give you the gift of time to take care of your family as best you can.

We know intellectually that we need to plan for the future, but since it means talking about our own death, it seems that we all put that planning off. We shouldn't. It's not a fun topic to deal with, but especially when faced with a tough diagnosis, you just can't put it off any longer. The future is now. That means that wills need to be drawn up or fine-tuned. Documents need to be gathered, things like insurance papers, deeds, notes about where things are located, or who can be counted on to help. It's a great idea to help those left behind by organizing some ideas about what they euphemistically call your "final disposition." It's a good idea to take care of any of the little details you can attend to now, so that in the terrible event that you don't beat this thing, you'll have helped to ease your family's burden. My family. My friends. My law practice. God, there was so much to be done. I knew that I needed a lot more time.

In that summer after the Gamma Knife, while we were waiting for the vaccine, and I was trying not to get too sucked into stress at the office, it became ever more important to keep my focus on what was really important. Gerri helped tremendously by running interference, helping me stay focused on family and on getting well.

Help Your Patient Get His or Her Affairs in Order

Although it can be a difficult subject for an advocate to broach, it's important to encourage your patient to make sure that he or she has legal and/or estate-planning documents in order. You can go on the Internet and find some standardized wills and other documents, but I think you should meet with an attorney who specializes in estate planning. Help your patient gather together all the documents an attorney will need to look at, such as home deeds, insurance papers, how his or her IRA is held—any and all documents that must be incorporated into an estate plan. And don't be fooled into thinking that an estate plan is just for someone with lots of money. Spending some time and effort right now can help save much of whatever you have saved for your loved ones, rather than leaving it for the tax man.

Have your patient talk to the human resources person at work and ask questions like, "Do I have disability insurance? Does our state pay any disability payments to me? If I wind up completely unable to work, does Social Security help?" An attorney will be able to help you find these answers, and I have also found that some hospitals have social workers who can help get these answers as well.

Gerri

I have to admit that there were times when it seemed that everything I was dealing with was more than I could handle. I had been doing my best to keep life as normal as possible, trying to keep our corner of the world as stress free as I could. And then the medical bills began to arrive. The number listed under the category of "amount due" was often staggering, and in many respects, confusing. I thought we had great medical insurance and couldn't understand why we still owed these huge amounts! My first inclination was to just pay the bills. After all, I had worked hard to find the best possible care for Brian, and the last thing I wanted to do was to get us in trouble with a medical provider by not paying a bill as soon as it arrived. I spent hours and hours trying to figure out Brian's medical bills, and hope that what I learned will save you from some of the problems I had.

Advocate Tip
#30

Pay Attention to the Medical Bills

You've been dealing with one incredibly difficult situation after another, and then they hit you again, this time from a different angle. The medical bills begin to arrive. With all that's going on in your life, there is a tendency to simply pay the bill no matter how huge the amount. After all, you've worked so hard to find the best possible care for your patient; the last thing you want is to get into trouble for not paying a bill. In reality, though, those bills often do not need to be paid.

In today's world of managed health care (if you're lucky enough to be insured), it's likely that your insurance company has entered into a contract or agreement with the hospital, doctor, and/or other medical provider. As part of their contract, the medical providers agree to take whatever discounted amount the insurer has agreed to pay them.

You are often *not* responsible for the difference between the amount charged and the contracted amount, even though you receive a bill from the provider with a message in big, block red letters: "Your insurance company has paid its share of the bill. You are responsible for the remainder." Incorrect!

If this happens, call your insurance company and ask, Has my medical provider entered into a contract with you to accept a certain amount? If so, can they charge me for the remainder of the amount? Once you have that information in hand, call your medical provider and tell them what you've learned. Every time I did this, I was told, "Oh, gosh. You're absolutely correct. That's just a billing error!" Sometimes, it took several calls to the providers to straighten things out, but given the exorbitant amount of the bills, I was happy to call back. This is extremely important, as those bills are often very expensive and are capable of wiping out a family's financial resources in a heartbeat.

Another hint when it comes to paying bills: delay. When the bills start rolling in, don't even open them for a month. Just put them aside, all in one place for safekeeping. When you can find some quiet time, sit down with this as your project. First, take a deep breath and then open all the bills, sort them by provider, and put them in chronological order. Then wait until you have the insurance statements in hand and sort them chronologically, too, before you attempt to pay any "patient responsibility" amounts. The delay will give you the time you need to make certain that you're not overpaying.

Seeing medical bills with their mind-boggling amounts can cause anyone to lose sleep, but I believe the peace of mind gained by handling things is well worth the effort. At the end of every bill-paying session, I recommend that you pour yourself a glass of wine, eat some chocolate, or relax in the bathtub. You will have earned it!

If you think it's more than you can handle in this difficult time, ask someone you can rely on to handle the bills for you. There are also for-profit companies that will review records for medical billing errors and work to correct insurance-billing mistakes. See page 213.

Another major aspect of patient finances concerns insurance coverage. Because we were fortunate and had no difficulty with coverage, I haven't had much personal experience with this nightmare, but I know that many have. Sometimes insurance companies will deny that they need to cover a given treatment, especially if they consider that treatment "experimental." Or if they provide coverage, the company may put a cap on the amount they'll pay. If you are not able to get the relief you need from an insurance company on your own, try contacting your state insurance department. The Patient Advocate Foundation, a nonprofit advocacy group, has volunteer attorneys who might also be able to help. For more information about this group, see page 213.

Brian

Gerri's taking care of so many of the stressful details of managing my illness helped me to turn my attention to what mattered to me. Despite my general optimism that I would make it through the illness, I wanted my kids, and eventually their kids, to have an understanding of some of the things I had done, things I had experienced, what I had learned, and more important, the mistakes I had made. Kathi and Patrick had lived in a different world from mine, and I wanted to impart to them my experience to use if and when they chose. There was so very much I had seen, lived, and learned. Even more significantly, I wanted to express the feelings that we had shared over the years.

In the beginning, all I had was a title, *Dad's Gift*. Since I really didn't know how to begin this project, I started by compiling lists. First came a list of poetry that had been important to me, followed by a list of the books that meant so much to me during my life. During my years at sea with the navy, and for several years thereafter, I had kept a journal that included things I had written myself or quotes from books I had read. I included parts of this journal in the book I was creating for the kids. As I began to write, a flood of memories came washing through me: the laughter long forgotten; the mistakes I'd made as both a child and an adult, many of which still haunted me; my childhood dreams; the complicated decisions I'd made; and so many books I felt must be read. In short, my life's great passions. The writing of *Dad's Gift* became cathartic.

When Kathi and Patrick were kids, I tried every night to tell them a new fairy tale of my own invention. It had been a very special part of their young lives and something I really enjoyed. Now, it was my hope they would be able to pass this storytelling along to their children. With that in mind, I came up with a guide that described how to create one's own fairy tales. I called this "Brian's Do-It-Yourself Fairy Tale Kit" (see page 218 for details).

The heritage of the Irish includes the telling of tales and the singing of songs, and I've done my share of both. Sure now, how could I not include my favorite Irish jokes? I also included lists of my favorite movies, songs, and quotations. I then sat down with Kathi and Patrick separately, and asked each of them to share some of their most vivid memories of childhood. I also added some of my memories about my mother and dad, both of whom had died in the 1980s, and included a story called "Moments That Make the Man," which charted significant memories of my early years.

Because the legal profession had been such a significant part of my life, I wrote a section called "A Life in the Courtroom." Like any single parent who also tried to juggle a professional life, I carried the burden of "maybe I should have been there more than I was." Finally, I talked about cancer and my reactions to it.

A year later, I would revise *Dad's Gift* and give it to Mark and Todd, having included individual stories for them from their childhoods. In all, it was a fulfilling process that I enjoyed enormously. The writing of memories, thoughts, and experiences brought me a sense of clarity. I would encourage everyone, whether facing serious illness or not, to take the time to record important memories and thoughts. It can be a wonderful gift to give your children and their children.

Make Memories and Share Stories

Support your loved one in making a record of his life for his family. Although it can be awkward, don't hesitate to take out your camera or video camera during family gatherings, trying your best not to create any pressure about recording moments "for posterity." You don't need to make a big deal of it, but family and friends will be very glad to have a record of the good times, whatever the future holds.

While Brian needed no prompting to smile for a camera, or tell his stories and share his "gift," others might. Encourage your patient to use whatever media he's comfortable with—whether videotape, scrapbooks, or journals—to share the highlights of his life with those he may leave behind.

Brian

Over the past ten years, our family has grown significantly. My children have had children, and so have Gerri's. Between us, we have seven wonderful grandchildren, who sure know how to keep us focused on what's important. In many ways, this new generation of children is the core of our new life, and the center of our new focus. Once again, it was Gerri who took the lead in making sure that we are very involved in their lives. It has brought me immeasurable happiness to watch Gerri with our grandkids. She has pitched hours of batting practice to them and gone camping with them under sheets strung between chairs (excuse me, "forts"). She spends far more time and energy looking for clothes for the girls than she ever does for herself, and plays cards and games with them by the hour. Our grandchildren have given us more joy than we thought possible. As someone once told us, "Having grandchildren is one of the few things in life that is not overrated." What's more, I believe that I have a special sense of appreciation for the experience. I know I could have missed it all.

Chapter Seven

KEEP ON FIGHTING

If you're going through hell, keep going.
—WINSTON CHURCHILL

Gerri

"**B**rian, can you say your name?"

When I go back and look at my reactions to certain events, they often seem bizarre. My initial response to having my husband look at me and babble incoherently certainly fits into that category. It was a few days before Thanksgiving, 1998. I'd just asked Brian where he wanted to take his cousin to lunch. Brian was looking at me and, in mid-sentence, his speech became completely nonsensical. It wasn't as if he was just mixing up words; this was more like a combination of sounds that didn't mean anything at all.

As he sat in front of me making these incoherent sounds, I asked him, over and over, to say his name. I even gave him a hint. "*Brian*, can you say your name?" He couldn't. Perhaps this was simply my way of stalling until *my* brain could figure out how to react. Brian could walk and move his arms and legs, which made me think that he wasn't having a stroke, but I didn't have a clue as to what the problem was. I stayed as calm as I could, but my heart was in my throat. Having the person you love look at you while speaking in tongues evokes a terrifying feeling.

By the time I drove Brian to the emergency room, his speech was almost back to normal, although he had trouble focusing on words and his memory was shaky. He seemed to be totally exhausted. He was immediately given CT scans, which showed no obvious signs of any problems other than the two brain tumors, which were still evident. The emergency room doctor ordered the steroid Decadron, and told us to contact our neurosurgeon.

Brian

"Where do you want to take your cousin for lunch?" Gerri asked.

Sitting on the edge of our bed, I leaned over to tie my shoelaces and then came back up and answered her question. At least, in my mind, I answered her question. Unfortunately, it sounded like total gibberish.

It was several months since I'd been weaned off my initial round of steroids. Now we know that we were dealing with a small focal brain seizure, but at that time, all Gerri knew was that within sixty seconds she had seen me go from speaking normally to sounding like a Martian.

The lady in the yellow tennis dress took over, and without so much as a gasp, Gerri was at my side. As far as I know, all my previous encounters with speaking in tongues had been Bushmills-driven, and the nonsense coming out of my mouth now should have been enough to send Gerri running from the room in a panic. I've decided that in a former life, she must have been a doctor or a medic or a four-star general—someone trained to be calm in the face of a crisis. She insists that it's simply a function of being the oldest of six kids.

She sat down next to me. "Bri, I think that we may need to get some medication for you. I just want you to try and relax and rest for a minute while I get dressed and then I'm going to drive us to the hospital."

Since it was early on a Saturday morning, Gerri took me to the emergency room. They did a CT scan of my brain, and the emergency room doctor recommended putting me on intravenous steroids. Gerri spent a lot of time telling him my medical background and also told him of my hyper reaction to steroids at the 10-mg level. This doctor nodded, and after completing his examination, he left the room.

Soon after, a nurse came in and was about to inject something into the intravenous line they had started when Gerri asked to see the label to see what I was being given. It was steroids, but at twice the level Gerri had warned was a problem for me. Since it was going to be administered right into my bloodstream in combination with the pills I had previously taken, it would have had an even stronger effect. Gerri told the same story to the nurse that she had told the doctor, but this time it was different. The woman actually listened and ran for the doctor, who by that time had left. While we waited, Gerri looked at the intravenous line and told me that she figured she could clamp it off. If we had to, we would simply do that, remove the IV, and leave. The nurse returned and told us she hadn't been able to reach the doctor. Gerri told her that we were leaving, with or without her help. The nurse smiled. "If I were in your position I'd be doing the exact same thing," she said. She helped us remove the IV and we were on our way.

Ask Questions—Constantly

This is one area in which Brian and I believe that the role of an advocate is vital. Your patient is going to be at the mercy of medical personnel who are often overworked and underpaid. A July 2006 report issued by the Institute of Medicine (an arm of the National Academy of Sciences) had the foreboding title "Preventing Medication Errors." The report estimated that there are at least 400,000 preventable injuries and deaths in hospitals each year due to medication errors. A July 2004 study by Health Grades, a health care ranking agency, concluded that nearly 200,000 people *die* each year due to "preventable hospital medical errors." That's nearly a quarter of a million people who die each year—while in hospitals—a quarter of a million people who die in *preventable* hospital accidents. If hospital error were listed as a leading cause of death in our country, it would rank in sixth place—ahead of diabetes, pneumonia, and Alzheimer's.

Far too many mistakes are made in hospitals and even physicians' offices by medical personnel who are unable to read the doctor's written orders, or who are simply worn out and just make mistakes. Whatever the cause, your Brian may very likely be unable to check on his own medication. Your patient is unlikely to be in a position to question the need for a specific medication. And even when our loved ones have those capabilities, because they are now patients, they are unlikely to assert themselves. Most people who have been put in this situation have told me the same thing; they had placed themselves completely in the hands of the medical profession, and were unwilling to challenge medical personnel. Even the most competent person is unlikely to assert himself in this setting.

In many instances, it will be up to the advocate to ask those questions. Questions such as:

- What is that medication?
- What is it for?
- Does it work well with the other medications he/she is taking?
- What amount are you giving?
- What's the normal amount?
- What reactions should I be looking for?

When talking about treatment options, ask just as many questions. The day I asked a doctor a question and his response was "You're getting too much information off the Internet" was the last time we saw that physician. Competent, capable physicians are not threatened by someone who has information. They might have to tell you that your information is half baked, but they won't be threatened by it. Ask them:

- Have you done this treatment/procedure before? How many times?
- Who do you consider to be the best in this field?
- Why are you choosing this treatment as opposed to any other?
- What are the pluses and minuses?
- What are the chances this treatment will work?
- How will we know if it's working?
- What are the side effects of the treatment?
- If this treatment doesn't work, will it prevent us from trying other treatment options?
- Do you know of any clinical trials we could take part in?

Initially, you may not even know what the correct answers to most of these questions should be. But while you're on the road to discovering the answers, you'll have done something very important. You will have alerted the medical personnel that you are there, interested in what they are doing, and that you are willing to assert yourself and ask questions. You will have let them know that even though your patient cannot stand up for him- or herself, someone can. You can. Use whatever style works best for you. Be dominant or meek. Be hostile or ingratiating. Above all, let them know that someone is there, vigilant and caring.

I take it as a given that people who have chosen a medical career have done so because they really want to be in a position to help people. That nurse or doctor or therapist is not trying to kill your patient or cause harm in any way. But the statistics are frightening. Accidents do happen, so don't be too shy to question what's happening to your patient. And remember: just being in your patient's corner is one more item in the list of checks and balances that may well prevent harm from occurring.

Finally, don't forget to *write it all down*. Pull out that notebook you've been carrying around and use it. If you write down the words the doctor is telling you, even if you don't understand what he or she is saying at the time, you can always get help later in determining what they mean.

I think they made Gerri sign some form saying that we had declined treatment and we were out of there. Gerri had already put in a call to Mike McDermott. She knew that we would get better advice from someone who was more familiar with my situation. Within an hour, Dr. McDermott returned her call and immediately prescribed a dosage of steroids that would work for me.

Over the next few days, I had more MRIs of the brain and numerous conversations with the doctors up in San Francisco. Dr. McDermott called, saying he had some good news and some not so good news. I'm a sucker for this line and I gobbled up the good news first. First, there were no new tumors, which was great. Second, the smaller tumor, the one over the occipital lobe, was shrinking to the point where it was less than half the size it had been before, which was really great. Then the bad news. The large tumor over the left temporal lobe was about the same size as it had been, and there was definite swelling over the language cortex. This was not such good news.

The swelling explained my attempt to start a new language. Dr. McDermott went on to say that because six months had now passed since the Gamma Knife treatment, the swelling was likely the result of one of two things: it was either a persistent tumor, or trauma resulting from the Gamma Knife radiation therapy itself. Either way, it wasn't good.

Gerri

The doctors asked us to come to San Francisco so Brian could have a PET scan, which they described as the gold standard of scans since it would be able to determine if the tumor was still "alive" and active. Brian and I had already accepted the fact that whatever the cause, this was a problem we were just going to have to deal with. We were pretty nonchalant. At least as nonchalant as you can be about a brain tumor. We were under the assumption that we would just have to go back in for another Gamma Knife, and we already knew it was something we could handle pretty easily.

Unfortunately, this wasn't the case. When we met with the UCSF team, the doctors told us that a repeat Gamma Knife over the same area was not recommended. The only way to proceed would be to do an open craniotomy, and because of the location of the tumor, over his speech and language center, Brian would have to be *awake* during the operation. He would need to help the surgeons—to guide them—as they attempted to avoid irreparable damage to his ability to communicate.

Hearing this was almost as bad as hearing the words "brain tumors" for the first time. We were both blindsided and sat in stunned silence. Once again, the taste of bile rose in my throat. In a matter of moments, we had gone from thinking that dealing with this latest problem was going to be a cakewalk to realizing that Brian might need brain surgery—something we had been more than happy to avoid back in June.

We spent the next few hours telling each other that we'd been incredibly lucky so far and there was no reason to believe that this luck wouldn't continue. I held on to Brian, telling him it was going to be fine. But I had to keep swallowing to keep down that awful taste in my mouth.

After more CT scans and lab tests, we went home to wait for the results. As always, waiting was one of the most difficult times for me. The seemingly endless period of time when there aren't any answers is almost as bad as getting really terrible news. To make matters worse, in the midst of all this we got a call from Baylor. Dr. Banchereau was very excited: they had received final approval from the FDA and thought they were almost ready to begin the vaccine program. Now we had to tell them we weren't. We had waited for months for Baylor to be ready, and our one fear was that the brain tumors would come back and prevent Brian from entering their program. And now something was going on inside his brain but no one seemed to know what it was.

Gold standard or not, the PET scan was not conclusive. Finally, in mid-December, Dr. McDermott called and told us to reduce the dosage of the steroids Brian had been taking since the seizures in late November, in order to figure out what was going on. He said that if the rim of that one tumor was still active, this reduction would result in swelling of the area over the left temporal lobe. Radically reducing the steroid dosage would cause Brian to again experience "word problems and confusion" and reveal that the tumor, and not damage from the Gamma Knife surgery, was indeed the culprit.

It was not a particularly happy Christmas. In fact, it was the worst Christmas I can remember. Although we engaged in as much forced gaiety as we could, in reality, we were waiting for the other shoe to fall. It did on December 28th when Brian entered into one of those states of word confusion we have since learned to deal with. Brian couldn't add two simple numbers together and was having a great deal of difficulty making much sense at all. Because by now I had an idea of what to expect, I was able to deal with this somewhat more easily. But we now had the answer to what was causing this symptom, and it was a terrifying one. The rim of the tumor over the area that controlled all of his language capabilities was still active, and our only hope in dealing with it was the open craniotomy.

I called Mike McDermott and he scheduled the surgery for January 6, 1999.

Don't Schedule Surgery During the Holidays

Advocate Tip
#33

If it's not an absolute emergency, have surgery scheduled outside any normal holiday schedule. This is the time when many medical professionals take some vacation time. When I first spoke to Dr. McDermott, he told me that he could do Brian's surgery on January 2nd. I asked him if Brian's condition would allow him to wait another few days for the operation, and he replied it wouldn't cause a problem. Then I asked him if the A-team would be back from Christmas vacations by January 2nd.

He laughed. "I'll be there. That counts for something, right?"

I told him that we wouldn't want to go through this without him. But when I asked him again if the rest of the A-team would be there, there was a long pause. Then he said, "How about January 6th?" Dr. McDermott knew why I was pestering him. The rest of his A-team, the people with whom he regularly performed this surgery, who knew the procedure inside and out, would not be there on the 2nd. While I'm willing to believe that everyone in the medical field is wonderful, I also believe that just as in any other field, there is an A-team in medicine. I wanted to be sure that Brian had access to the best of the best. I wanted him to have the A-team. Make sure you ask for that team as well.

Brian

Neurosurgery is something no one wants. The prospect was terrifying. I was comfortable in the fact that we were dealing with the best doctors and staff we could have, and I knew that they would all be doing their best. But still, the problem was that the tumor rested directly adjacent to the speech and language portion of my brain. Any misstep would render me "significantly impaired." That was doctor-talk for the possibility that the Brian Monaghan I had been for sixty years would no longer exist. A pretty heavy thought. Speech and the ability to communicate—we all take these things for granted. I sure did. I had made my living in part by means of my skill as a speaker, convincing judges and juries with words, and now I faced the prospect that not only would I lose that skill completely, I might lose the ability to communicate on the most basic level.

During the summer, I had done everything concrete I could do in terms of wills, insurance papers, documents on hand, and taking care of things at the firm. I told the kids that there was no reason to believe that my luck was about to run out now. At night, I held Gerri as we reassured each other that I would be fine. But I was terrified. My biggest fear was that I would come out of this some sort of vegetable, with all my thoughts locked inside my body. To me, that didn't sound like much of a life. I reminded Gerri of our talks about not wanting to live in a persistent vegetative state, and she promised me that she would let them "pull the plug" if it ever got to that. As we write this book now, I get chills when I stop and recall how bad this period was for us.

The only good part was that we didn't spend time trying to decide whether or not I should have this surgery. I could either take the chance or quit. If I didn't have the operation, I'd be dead within months anyway. When certain death is your only option, I think the choice is pretty easy. Gerri and I began approaching the craniotomy with the attitude we had assumed before: let's get it done—we know it's going to succeed. At least, that's what we said to each other. I don't think either one of us believed it completely.

Gerri and I arrived at UCSF a day or two before the surgery and spent lots of time going from one doctor's office to another. They each took a shot at letting me know what to expect. They told me I'd need to be awake during the surgery so they could utilize what is called "mapping," a procedure that would help them avoid the area that controlled my language cortex. This was one of the pluses of being at UCSF. They were one of the first places to have mapping technology, which showed them exactly how far down into the brain they needed to go. The doctors explained that I would be put under anesthesia while they were cutting through my skull, but that once they had cut out a section, I would be brought back up into kind of a twilight state. I would receive some medication but would still be awake. I accepted this. But accepting the *idea* of something and accepting the reality of that idea are two different things!

Gerri

The night before Brian's craniotomy, Steve and Susan Parker had come to San Francisco to offer moral support. By the time they arrived, Brian had already had the brain-mapping MRI, during which the radiology team had glued small, round sensors to several spots on his skull and over each of his eyebrows. They told us that Brian had to keep the sensors in place until the operation as they would be essential in helping guide doctors to the exact site of the brain tumors. These sensors weren't sinister looking at all, but they were very prominent. The four of us had already planned on going out to dinner that evening. After lots of laughing and kidding about Brian's weird appearance, we looked at each other, shrugged, and said, "Let's go eat." San Francisco being San Francisco, no one batted an eye at the man with the electrodes on his head as we had a poignant, often teary-eyed dinner together.

The next day, during our pre-dawn drive through the deserted streets of the city, we all took turns at nervous, meaningless chatter. As we walked through the nearly empty parking garage, I reached into my purse for some breath mints and offered one to Susan. She looked at them and squealed, "Look. They look just like the things on Brian's head." I'm not sure how it started—probably some kind of hysterical reaction to what we were facing—but by the time we got into the elevator, Susan, Steve, and I had each licked the back of two breath mints and had stuck them on our faces so we looked like Brian. Susan and I were cackling. The one other person riding along in the elevator reached over and pressed the button for the next floor. He couldn't get away from us fast enough!

We spent the next hour or so standing around Brian while he did his best to keep our spirits up. That's not a typo. Brian worked at keeping *our* spirits up and, as he often did, he accomplished that through humor. A short time after we arrived, a nurse came into our cubicle and asked the Parkers to leave so Brian could change into the flimsy hospital gown. When they were allowed back in, Susan pointed at Brian and began laughing. I hadn't realized it, but under the cover of the sheet, Brian had raised his index finger in a strategic place. There was no doubt he was telling us that he was facing the day with unbridled enthusiasm. Facing the possibility of surgery that could change him into a completely different person, Brian still had the amazing ability to keep us all upbeat. We did manage to laugh that morning, and when they came to get him, Brian gave me a kiss, a wave, and said, "See you later, kid!" As they wheeled him toward the operating room, I didn't know if he would come back as anything close to the man I loved.

Brian

For eight and a half hours I lay on my right side in surgery with my head pinned down to prevent even the slightest movement. The team shaved the hair on the left side of my head, then cut through the side of my skull. After that part of my skull was removed, it was put aside on a sterile field. Basically, my head was a Halloween pumpkin someone cuts the top off and places on a counter. Next came the difficult part as they went in after the tumor. A neuropsychologist sat in front of me, constantly asking me questions and showing me pictures to identify, all to determine if my cognitive brain functions were intact. The neuropsychologist would show me a picture of a helicopter and say, "Can you tell me what this is?" I felt like I was on *Sesame Street*.

Although I guess it wasn't funny at the time, a "Brian Monaghan moment" occurred in the middle of the surgery. During the meeting we had had with Dr. McDermott the day before, he had gone over all the legalities of the operation. One of the things he told us was that I had the right to stop the surgery at any time. It seemed highly unlikely to either Gerri or me that someone would get up and walk out of the room in the middle of brain surgery. We had all laughed.

Now, though, with my head cut open like a jack-o'-lantern and the surgeons getting ready to go after my tumor, I had a reaction to the local anesthesia they were using. I suddenly reached out and started pulling at the restraints, trying to get up off the table. Actually, my memory is that I reached out and grabbed the anesthesiologist, but that may just be what I wanted, and was trying my best, to do. I told Dr. McDermott, "Doctor, I'm getting the feeling that this is going nowhere. I want out of here!"

Everything came to a dead stop. Dr. McDermott said, "Get John back in here." John Walker was the neuropsychologist. With his face just inches from mine, he calmly talked to me, telling me that I had gotten overly apprehensive due to the medication. He told me that the surgery had been stopped and would not continue until I gave the word. He told me that he would attempt to regulate the anesthesia to make me more comfortable, and once we reached that point, I could make the decision as to whether I wanted to proceed or not. His calm words and the change in medication must have worked, as I obviously reached the conclusion that it made no sense to try and put the side of my head back on until they dealt with the tumor. I told them they could go ahead.

Ten years later, Dr. McDermott still shakes his head at my attempt to escape brain surgery.

Gerri

D r. McDermott had promised that he would keep me updated on the progress of the surgery and he was true to his word. Every hour I received a call from someone in the operating room, telling me that everything was "proceeding smoothly" and that Brian was doing fine. At 4:15, just about eight hours after they had wheeled Brian into the OR, Mike McDermott called to say the operation had gone well: Brian was talking to everyone; his motor functions were intact; his cognitive functions appeared to be normal as well. Dr. McDermott then went on to tell me about Brian trying to get off the operating table. He said that it had been pretty tense for a while, especially when Brian's brain had literally swelled up into the opening. McDermott and his assistant reached over, spread out their hands, and slowly pushed the brain back down. What an image!

The agonizing wait was over. The Parkers and I hugged one another, each of us reacting to this wonderful news in our own way. I cried a little, but held most of it in until later. Susan cried a lot. And Steve muttered something like, "That SOB just does this stuff to get extra attention!" I got on the phone to share the good news with all the kids and also started the phone tree to pass on the news to everyone.

Within an hour, I had talked my way into the post-surgical intensive care unit—it was an unbelievable experience. When he saw me, Brian gave a big smile, a wave, and a "Hi, Ger!" as if he had just returned from a day at the office. He was amazing. His words were clear, as was his recognition of people, names, and objects. He didn't seem to be in any pain, and other than the huge bandages on his head and all the tubes coming in and out of his body, it was hard to tell that he had undergone this incredibly difficult procedure. But it had been tough. My guy, who can handle anything (except the common cold), told me that the experience of being awake and semi-lucid throughout eight hours of brain surgery was something that he didn't think he could ever go through again.

Be There

Advocate Tip
#**34**

Whenever your patient is hospitalized, you as the advocate need to be right by his or her side. It is so important to maintain as much of a presence as you can. Not only for your patient, but simply to be "the presence"—the one they are probably talking about at the nurses' station. You might find some medical staff who will make you feel as if you're in the way, but everyone who's worth his salt knows how important it is to have a vigilant advocate by the patient's side. It's just too easy for something to go wrong.

How much of a presence should you maintain? While I advocate being at the bedside 24/7, and truly admire those caregivers who do it, I can't. I am one of those people who need a fairly good night's sleep to function well the next day. I can "camp out" on a chair next to Brian's bedside for a night, maybe two, but that's about it. Early on, I had to make the decision that there was only so much I could do. Only so much energy I had. Only so much that I could take physically, as well as mentally. I need sleep, and if that meant leaving Brian alone in the hospital from midnight to six in the morning, that's what I had to do. Everyone has different tolerance levels, but the important thing is to be there in the hospital with your patient as much as *you* can.

By 8:00 the next morning they had dismissed Brian from the ICU (Brian's humor is infectious, and they told him they needed the bed for someone who was *really* sick). After a good-size breakfast he was back in a regular room, and within a few hours he'd showered and was up and around the hallways doing his "Monaghan walk," charging full speed ahead. Nurses assigned him an aide, but since the man was about 5 feet 5, he had little chance of keeping up with Brian, and after a few loops around the perimeter, he just gave up and let Brian go on his own with me trailing not too far behind.

Brian was euphoric and I was, too. The idea of losing the Brian I loved had been agonizing, and I have developed great empathy for those who are faced with the thought of losing someone to Alzheimer's or other types of brain damage. We are just so grateful to the UCSF team that he came through this with such great success.

The doctors told me that Brian's mental acuity and ability to speak immediately after the surgery would be the best indicator of how he had come through, but that within twenty-four hours, the brain would swell again in response to the trauma of the surgery. When this happened, his speech, memory, and cognitive functions would regress until days later when the swelling subsided. They were right. It was like clockwork. Within twenty-four hours Brian couldn't name simple objects, like a clock or a flashlight. He couldn't read any numbers, or give the names of our children or our dog. He couldn't remember his own birth date but instead, kept insisting to the nurse that he was thirty years old. Still, in one of those cruel little tricks of fate, when the nurse asked him all these questions, he would just point to me and say "1944." He couldn't remember his own birthday, but he had the nerve to remember the year in which I was born! The nurses loved it.

How to Live Through a Hospital Experience

Advocate Tip
#**35**

During the past ten years, I have spent way too much time in hospitals. But in that time, I have come to learn a great deal about how the advocate can make their patient's hospital stay better. Like most people, Brian hates being in hospitals. He doesn't mind the surgery, or the recovery, or the pain involved, but having to stay in a hospital room makes him a truly unhappy camper. The following ideas—some my own, some from other advocates, some gleaned from doctors and nurses, some grand and some picayune—will all help:

- **First rule: Get out of there as soon as possible!**
- **Don't schedule surgery during the holidays** (see Tip #33, page 110).
- **Avoid teaching hospitals in the summer months** when the new interns have just made their way into hospital life. I know that they're there to learn, but my philosophy is to let them practice on someone else!
- **Don't take no as a final answer** (see Tip #36, page 122).
- **Find out when your best chance to see the doctor is.** The doctors usually do their hospital rounds (visits to patients) very early in the morning. Ask the nurse when it is that your particular doctor is usually seen on your floor. Whatever that time is, if you need to speak with the doctor personally as opposed to getting information secondhand from the patient, you need to be there. If it's 7:00 a.m., set your alarm early

and be there—or spend a night by your patient's bedside and surprise the doctor in the morning! This is a twofer as it will remind them that someone is there who is vitally interested and ever-watchful.

• **Find out when the physical or occupational therapist will be working with your patient**, and make sure you're there as well. There's a strong chance that your patient will be groggy and unable to remember exactly what he or she was told to do. If you observe the therapy session, you can remind your patient later.

• **Make friends with everyone!** From the doctors to the nurses' aides to the woman pushing the mop around the room—if they like you, they will go the extra mile for you. Treat them each as a valuable member of the team trying to help your patient, because in reality, they are (see Tip #40, page 139).

• **Make certain that everyone who enters your patient's room washes his or her hands.** We all know that germs are often spread on contact and we've heard of staph infections that can spread through hospitals. The November 2008 AARP Bulletin contained an article by Betsy McCaughey, a former lieutenant governor of New York, about a lesser-known bacteriuim that is also extremely virulent. *"C. diff"* (*Clostridium difficile*) has infected thousands of patients, and the last part of its Latin name indicates how bad this superbug is. Antibacterial soaps (often found on the wall of every patient room) won't kill it, and the only way to stop it is by having everyone entering a patient's room thoroughly wash his or her hands with soap and water. McCaughey said that before eating anything, patients should wash their hands as well. Because clothing can also carry the bug, she recommended that contact with hospital restaurants be avoided and that all clothing brought home be washed separately. Ask your hospital what steps they are taking—and what steps you can take—to help your patient avoid hospital infections. The people treating your patient are all trained to wash their hands when they enter a patient's room, and also prior to leaving. Make sure they do it. If they don't, you need to remind them of this practice. You can be "nice" about it or just matter-of-fact, but make sure it's done as it can help save your patient from serious illness and even death.

• **Be there 24/7, or as much as you can** (See Tip #34, page 115).

• **Bring comforts from home** (See Tip #37, page 123).

- **Find out where the nurses' station kitchen is.** Find out where the juice, Jell-O, and water are kept, and once you're clear about any possible dietary restrictions for your patient, get those things yourself. Not only will your patient appreciate it, but the overworked nurses and aides will appreciate being freed up to provide the real medical assistance they are trained to provide. It's another twofer.
- **Find out where the linen closet is** and get any extra bed pads or blankets or pillows that your patient needs. Help make your patient as comfortable as possible by not having them wait for these things.
- **Help with bathroom assistance.** It may take too long for a nurse's aide to arrive to help with a urinal, so provide that assistance yourself. Another detail: on the side of the urinal you'll find numbers that indicate fluid output. Before emptying it out, make note of the amount and then write that number down. When the nurses aide shows up just prior to shift change with a look of panic, frantic with the thought that the patient hasn't urinated all day, you'll be able to provide the information needed to fill out the chart.
- **Be extra careful and vigilant around the time of shift changes.** Some hospitals are now on twelve-hour shifts, while others are on the normal eight-hour shifts. Find out what your hospital is on, and then make it a point to be there around that time. I have found that there's often a void in care during this time frame. The departing staff is busy preparing the charts and the arriving staff spends lots of time reviewing that information. It's a good time to be at the bedside and on the alert.

Brian

It was amazing how quickly I recovered from the craniotomy. Within seventy-two hours of the surgery, I was released from the hospital. Gerri and I stayed in San Francisco for a few days, and during that time my earlier confusion began to improve. I had some residual headaches, but really felt pretty good.

When it came to what I looked like—not so good! I was due to accept an award from a nonprofit I was involved in, the American Ireland Fund, at a fund-raiser in San Diego at the end of February. So prior to the operation, Gerri had talked the doctors into shaving only half my head in the hope that somehow

I would look better that way. This was one of the few times I can say she was wrong. Really wrong. If you saw me from the right side, everything looked fine, but if I turned my head just slightly, it looked as if the left side of my head had been scalped.

The doctors had explained to us that if just one single cancer cell broke loose during the operation, it would likely cause another tumor, and in their efforts to eliminate that possibility they had lined the surgical cavity where the tumor had been with little pellets of nuclear radiation. Because of that, I now had to wear a ridiculous looking, lead-lined helmet to protect everyone else from being exposed to unwanted radiation. I took this very seriously as my daughter, Kathi, was pregnant and due with triplets in July, and our daughter-in-law, Sharon, was pregnant and due in September. Wearing the helmet, I looked like an alien, but the last thing I wanted was to expose anyone to unnecessary risks. The radiation pellets had a relatively quick half-life of about six weeks and at that point, I was told, I could get rid of the alien look.

All in all, I had nothing to complain about. I felt as if we had won another round in our battle and I came home with the attitude that we were ready to get on with the fight against the cancer itself. The doctors at Baylor told us that after receiving their approval from the FDA, they had incurred an unexpected delay but that they would soon be ready to begin the dendritic-cell vaccine.

When I found out that my brain surgery hadn't really affected my shot at the vaccine, I was charged up. Again we got permission from Dr. McDermott to begin coming off the steroids at a much faster pace than is usually recommended. This meant I would have to deal with a lot more headaches and fatigue, but I was insistent that we get going with the vaccine program. I was excited about taking this major step forward, but then I took a couple of steps back. Big steps.

About ten days after the brain surgery, I began to feel significant pain in my left leg. I told Gerri about it, and very uncharacteristically, she said that she didn't want to hear any more of my whining, that we had been through enough. I guess she was worn out by the whole ordeal. She thought it might be some sort of muscular problem from my lack of exercise.

In fact, one of the risks of the procedure I'd just undergone was that the body emits protective agents to create blood clots when there has been major trauma, e.g., surgery. Usually the clots occur within a day or so, and all the necessary precautions had been taken to make sure they didn't occur while I was in the hospital. We knew that blood clots were extremely dangerous—they could break loose and go to the heart, lungs, or brain (or whatever remained of my brain)—but since the "normal" period for the occurrence of clots had passed, we thought I was home free. But I guess I don't do things normally.

By the next day, I was in lots of pain and walking with a definite limp. Gerri called my longtime physician, who immediately became concerned because I had a history of phlebitis in that left leg. He sent me for an ultrasound, which showed a large clot going from the back of my knee up into the groin. When we got to our local hospital, they refused to admit me because I was carrying nuclear radiation pellets inside my head. I was left sitting in the lobby during what was a very dangerous period of time. That clot could have broken free as I sat there.

Once again, the need for a strong advocate became apparent. Gerri took over and demanded to see the head of nursing, the head of the hospital, and then used one of the phrases left over from her years as a paralegal. She told the admissions people, "You ought to notify your carrier."

Gerri

By the time I came around to understanding that Brian's problem was a blood clot, I knew that we were dealing with something dangerous enough to kill him on the spot. That the spot could have been a hospital lobby was absolutely unacceptable to me. We filled out the paperwork for admissions and waited. And waited.

I tried sitting there patiently. But I knew how serious things were. I began going up to the desk, and as nicely as I could,

121

asked why Brian had not yet been admitted. They kept telling me that no rooms were available. Then, during one of my trips to the front desk, someone slipped and mentioned their concern that the radiation pellets that had been implanted in Brian's brain might "leak" to other patients. The admissions people had somehow decided that they were not going to take the chance and admit him. Since this happened on the Martin Luther King holiday (don't emergencies usually happen on nights, weekends, or holidays?), I couldn't immediately reach his doctors who could confirm to them my explanation that the radiation was under control by dint of Brian's special lead-lined helmet.

I understood the staff's concerns, but as always, my focus was on getting Brian the care he needed. Any thought of being nice ended for me at the moment I understood they were having us wait for nothing. I demanded to see the head of nursing, the head of admissions, and the head of the hospital. And I did tell them that I was putting the hospital on notice that if anything serious happened to Brian because of their failure to admit him, they would be held responsible.

Miraculously, somehow, almost instantaneously, a private room became available. I'm sure they thought I was a bitch from hell, but I didn't care. Brian was going to get the care he needed.

Advocate Tip
#36

Don't Take No as Their Final Answer

There is a time to accept what medical professionals tell you and a time to assert yourself on behalf of your patient. If you believe your patient needs something that's being denied her, I strongly recommend pushing for what is needed. No matter what kind of resistance you meet, you always have legal recourse, and reminding hospitals and doctors' offices of this can be an effective last resort.

Brian

I'd be lying if I told you that I never lost my positive attitude. It's easy to sometimes get down in your fight against cancer, or heart disease, or Parkinson's, or whatever else it is that you are facing down as an opponent. There were many times when I had to remind myself that it's really not just a battle. It's a war, and it often seems as if it goes on and on.

Whenever I got down, I deliberately tried to refocus my thoughts on something else. When I was told that I needed an open craniotomy, there's no denying that I sat there feeling sorry for myself. But a few minutes later, they wheeled a boy of about ten past us and we saw that his head was encased inside what we recognized as the Hannibal Lecter mask of the Gamma Knife. The thought that this young child was dealing with a brain tumor was the slap of reality I needed. It made me feel like a total wuss. I thought about what a great life I had lived for the past sixty years, while he might never get the same chance. That was something to really feel sorry about.

I found that it was often easier for me to deal with the major problems that arose while the small stuff could drive me crazy. Dealing with those blood clots was a case in point. I walked out of a hospital less than seventy-two hours after the top of my skull had been sitting next to me, yet blood clots kept me completely confined to a hospital bed for a week!

Bring the Comforts of Home

Whenever Brian was hospitalized, I did everything I could think of to make him as comfortable and as happy as possible. I brought photos of our family. I brought cards made by our grandchildren and taped them to his walls. Just as soon as he was able to get out of a hospital gown, I brought in his own pajamas, bathrobe, and slippers. A nurse told me that this was a big waste of time as I would have to take them home and launder them, but I think that's a small price to pay to give someone a feeling of comfort. I'm convinced that every little bit helps. During Brian's later hospitalizations, Steve Parker always showed up with a small DVD player and movies. And I would bring Brian audio books and some of his favorite music to help pass the time.

Like everyone else who is hospitalized, he complained mostly about the food. After his first hospitalization, it dawned on me that there wasn't really any reason for him to eat that food. I checked with the nurses to see what his dietary restrictions were, and taking that into account, I brought him dinner from restaurants in the area. Often, when the restaurant heard I was bringing food to my husband who was in the hospital, we would find extra goodies in the bag. Beyond the food itself, every morning I brought in some knives and forks, even napkins. Brian thought that this was all very "froufrou-ey," but he never turned it down.

When Brian felt well enough, I got the word out to friends. When someone asked me what they could do to help, I said, "Bring dinner." Sure enough, friend after friend brought everything from Chinese to Italian. Often, these dinners became all-out parties with the nurses coming in several times to tell us to hold it down. One evening, as I was cleaning up from our "dinner party," one of the nurses said, "You guys sure enjoy life!" Obviously, she was right. We continued to focus on fighting this battle with love and laughter, with some of the comforts of home thrown in for good measure.

Brian

A month after the craniotomy, in February of 1999, I was honored to receive the Heritage Award from the American Ireland Fund, a nonprofit charity that has raised millions of dollars with its credo, "Peace, Culture, Charity." The money goes to causes of all kinds in both the north and south of Ireland. I've been involved with this charity since its founding in the early 1980s; along with many others, I believe that the monies the Ireland Fund has pumped into Ireland, especially in the north, have played a major role in helping to bring peace to that country.

The dinner put together by the fund was far beyond any expectations I had. The year before, Gregory Peck had been honored, so I knew I was in good company. It turned out to be a spectacular event with more than 900 guests dressed in black tie and gowns arriving to the sound of wailing bagpipes. Todd and Jennifer had flown in from Denver, Mark and Sharon came down from Los Angeles, and of course Kathi and Tom and Patrick were there as well. Cousins and old friends were in attendance, as were former classmates from the Naval Academy. There were tables filled with attorneys, former clients, and of course, The Lads, who were present in full force. A video of my life was shown, which emphasized the good fights I'd fought as an attorney, and my love of family and friends.

This event brought together people from all parts of my life who expressed their feelings about me—to me. It was extraordinary to be present and hear what they had to say about how I'd touched them. It's really one of the best gifts the battle with cancer has given me. People said things that were wonderful, deeply personal, and more direct than I would have ever expected. I'd been struggling with having to end my law career and, of course, with being sick. But I came away from that evening with a great sense of peace. Having people tell you that they love you, sensing their true caring, warmth, and concern, is as good as it gets and it happens all too rarely.

I had a funny sense that if I died at that very moment, it would be okay. But more than that, hearing what I meant to others fueled my desire to live up to what they had all just said about me. I was a fighter. I had to keep on fighting.

Chapter Eight

EXPECT THE UNEXPECTED

When it is dark enough, you can see the stars.
—RALPH WALDO EMERSON

Brian

Dressed in a T-shirt and shorts, I sat on top of the covers of a hospital bed in Dallas, Texas. Doctors, nurses, and scientists lined the walls of the small room, all staring at me expectantly. Over in one corner was a cart containing the Code Blue equipment used to revive someone whose heart stops beating. Dr. Joe Fay had explained that while he didn't think that the dendritic-cell vaccine would have any adverse effects, since I was the very first patient to receive it, they just didn't know for sure. This equipment was an extra precaution. As we waited for the vaccine to be brought over from the laboratory, the room was filled with a strange combination of tension and excitement. As far as I was concerned, my long wait was finally coming to an end. I wasn't afraid, just anxious to get started.

For Gerri and me, the wait to get the vaccine treatment had seemed never-ending. It had been nine months since Dr. Zanetti had first learned about the dendritic-cell vaccine and made it his mission to find it for me. It had been eight months since we had first met with Dr. Fay and he indicated that the program was close to securing FDA approval. Enormously difficult work had gone into getting the vaccine ready. It had been years in the making. The Baylor team had decided to go with eighteen patients in Phase One of this clinical trial. Counting the forty patients who were already in similar programs in Germany and Switzerland, there would be fewer than sixty people in the world who were receiving this vaccine.

From the time we had decided that this program gave me the best shot at living, we'd experienced a seemingly endless series of starts and stops and delays that none of us had anticipated. Though I was convinced that this program was "the one," Gerri had used the waiting period to do research to check out other programs. Nothing appeared to offer as much hope as Baylor.

No matter how hard you try, keeping up your spirits isn't always easy. There were times in those past ten months when Gerri's talk about pushing the envelope didn't seem so confident. I know my optimism plummeted each time we got a call from Baylor telling us that the start of the program had been delayed yet again. And I know that Gerri was terrified that we would be cut from the program each time she had to pick up the phone to report to the team that I had experienced another medical setback. But we had all hung in there and now, finally, we were ready to go.

Gerri

It was clear that the issue of the brain tumors was in a league of its own, and all the doctors we had seen viewed the brain tumors and the underlying melanoma as almost two different problems. We'd attacked the tumors. Now, finally, we were going to use the dendritic-cell vaccine to go after the cancer itself.

I had learned a lot about dendritic cells and how they work from my research, and I understood how the vaccine was supposed to work in the following way. First, Brian would be given a drug that increased the number of his white blood cells. The program at Baylor called for taking out some of these "extra" blood cells through a fairly noninvasive method called "apheresis." His blood would be taken out of one arm, passed through a centrifuge where the white blood cells were spun off and collected, and then pumped back into the other arm. The collected white cells would be taken to the laboratory where the scientists would go to work.

The dendritic cells were to be grown in the presence of protein extracts, or antigens, which were obtained from melanoma cancer cells. This process would take several weeks, after which the dendritic cells that had been "loaded" with the melanoma antigens would be given to Brian through needle injections at points close to his lymph node system, i.e., close to the armpits and groin. The dendritic cells were then expected to help other cancer-fighting cells within his system recognize, attack, and destroy the lurking cancer cells.

In trying to translate all of this into terms we could understand, I gave the dendritic cells a face and personality. I decided that they looked like yellow, smiley-faced Pac-Men (if you're old enough to remember the first video games, you know what I'm talking about). In my scenario, these Pac-Men carried signposts describing the evil, horrible cancer cells. With these signs, the dendritic Pac-Men cells were telling the other cancer-fighting cells, "When you see these evil cancer antigens, recognize them for the evil things that they are, and destroy!" In essence, the Baylor program was a search-and-destroy mission.

Not perfectly accurate, but it put a face on our cancer problem and a face on the method we were going to use to beat it. We now truly had a plan in place that we hoped would defeat Brian's cancer.

Advocate Tip
#38

Put a Face on Your Disease

In the first few weeks of our battle, I had come up with a *Star Wars* theme for us to focus on in regard to the Gamma Knife. Now, with the dendritic-cell vaccine, I visualized smiley-faced Pac-Men directing traffic within Brian's immune system. While I knew that patients are often taught the concept of visualization in an effort to relieve them of chronic pain, I hadn't realized that this is a common technique for fighting illness, too.

Instinctively, Brian and I just knew that it was important to have an image of something to fight against. In his typical way, he saw what was happening in his body in terms of a battle of Good versus Evil. In this instance, the dendritic cells were good and the cancer was evil. Whenever he took any medication, Brian thought of it as something going into his bloodstream to attack those "cancer suckers." This imagery was even more potent for him than my happy-looking Pac-Men.

Whatever image you and your patient come up with, it's invaluable to put a face on the condition so your patient can also visualize exactly what his or her body needs to do to get better.

Brian

As I sat on the bed with everyone staring at me, I felt like an exhibit in a natural history museum. But then the vaccine itself was brought in by Jacques Banchereau and Karolina Palucka. The two doctors hand-carried it over to the hospital from their lab, in a little cooler packed with ice, and it's not an exaggeration to say that they carried the thing with an air of reverence. I had been waiting for nine months, none too patiently, for this vaccine to arrive. But at that moment, Gerri and I looked across the room at each other with the realization that these dedicated scientists had been working on, and waiting for, this particular moment for more than ten years.

For many of them, this could well be a moment of great significance in their long and often frustrating battle against cancer. Gerri and I have come to learn that in many ways, these two scientists and the wonderful team with whom they work have put their personal lives on hold, dedicating themselves to working on this vaccine. I really felt honored and privileged to be the first recipient of their hard work.

The room fell totally silent as the three subcutaneous injections were given by Dr. Fay, one in my arm and one in each of my thighs. As the last injection was given, everyone in the room broke into applause. Then we all waited.

And waited.

I had no sense of fear or even concern. I had complete faith and trust in these scientists and the vaccine, and so I was very calm. Not so Dr. Banchereau. He looked like a cat on a hot tin roof. Every few minutes, Jacques would say in his strong French accent, "Brian, do you feel anything? Anything at all?" (Okay, it was more like, "Brion, du u feel anyzing? Anyzing at all?") Once again, my need to lighten the mood took over. The next time Jacques repeated his question, "Brian, do you feel anything?" I looked at him and said, "Yes, I do."

Suddenly my right arm shot up into the air in the salute made famous by Peter Sellers in the movie *Dr. Strangelove*. The room erupted in laughter from everyone but Jacques. Joe Fay finally stopped laughing long enough to explain, "Jacques, that's from *Dr. Strangelove!*"

Jacques Banchereau has come to be a good friend, and in the past few years we have shared many stories, some great wine and food, and much laughter. I have enormous respect for his work as a research scientist, but that never stopped me from needling him. Several weeks later, during my second round of injections, Jacques brought two noted scientists visiting from Paris into my hospital room to meet me. As they approached, I jumped off the bed, knelt before Jacques, and began to kiss his hand. Then I looked to the astonished scientists and said, "I know this is silly, but Dr. Banchereau asks us all to do this whenever he arrives." The poor scientists did not know just what to make of me, and Gerri, as always, was left with the job of trying to explain my behavior.

Despite the concern on that first day of the injections, there was never a need for the Code Blue carts. We remained in the hospital for several hours on the first occasion, but only waited a short time after the remaining treatments. Afterward, we went to a movie, had a nice dinner, and headed back to San Diego early the next morning. There were times immediately following the injections when I had headaches and some chills, but these symptoms were expected and easily treated with Tylenol. In fact, I had an even milder reaction than the Baylor team had anticipated. My reactions were nothing compared to what anyone going through chemotherapy experiences. There were a series of four more injections spread out over the course of the next few months, and I continued to be monitored and tested constantly.*

*For Dr. Jacques Banchereau's perspective as a research scientist, see page 209.

Gerri

In early August, we got a phone call from Dr. Banchereau to tell us that they had "very exciting news." Throughout the summer, Brian had continued to receive "all clears" from the MRIs and CT scans. Now Dr. Banchereau and Dr. Palucka told us that the blood testing had demonstrated a strong response from Brian's immune system, with an increase in both his "killer" cells and their "helper" cells. We were overjoyed, and after sharing the news with the kids and all of our closest friends, we broke out the bottle of Champagne I had been saving for this moment and made a toast to Brian's heroic dendritic cells.

There was no sign of cancer. His immune system had rebounded.

We were now outside the immediate danger zone. Both Dr. Banchereau and Dr. Palucka felt that there had been a significant response, and not only were they happy for us, but they felt that they had made great strides forward with this vaccine program. A new lease on life was beginning. As Sol Price told Brian, "You're now living on God's time."

One year after the initial injections, we went back to Dallas for a series of booster injections and were happy to learn that Brian's immune system had produced even more and better dendritic cells than the previous year. While my imagery of this process continued to be full of little Pac-Men, Brian spoke of "those guys in there, killing those cancer suckers."

To say that we feel lucky, blessed, and privileged to have been part of this program is a vast understatement. We stay in touch with the people at Baylor, and whenever Brian or I can go anywhere to speak on their behalf, we do so with the feeling that we can never repay them.

Brian

More than five years after the experiment began, there is hope for cancer patients through dendritic cells. ODC Therapy, Inc., is a biotech company created from the work at Baylor that now produces and distributes customized cancer vaccines to individual patients throughout the world. This is the product of more than fifteen years of research and development, and I continue to feel honored to have been the first person to get the vaccine. When ODC was launched, Carol Robertson (another vaccine recipient and cancer survivor) and I were asked to attend the press conference and discuss the effects of the dendritic-cell vaccine. Carol's circumstances were very dramatic: her melanoma had been clearly visible as black spots on her legs. She had gone through the most radical chemotherapy imaginable, but it had been completely unsuccessful. The photos of her condition before and after the dendritic-cell vaccine were startling. After the vaccine, all the black spots on her legs disappeared. Carol and I happily agreed that by being part of this clinical trial, in our own small way we might be helping other cancer patients. I have continued to have MRIs and CT scans on a regular basis, but at the ten-year mark, I continue to show no signs of a recurrence of cancer. None!

In mid-April of 1999 Gerri had arranged for us to return to our yearly retreat in Puerto Vallarta, Mexico, and somehow managed to sandwich the vacation between vaccine treatments in Dallas. I was feeling pretty good about life at that point. It seemed as if I had come through the difficult part of dealing with the brain tumors without too much trauma. The vaccine program was finally in full swing and had been easy to handle. I was in full R & R mode as we were enjoying our time surrounded by good friends, enjoying a margarita or two, and soaking up the warmth and tranquillity of Ocho Cascadas, a place we both loved.

I have learned the hard way that often when I hit an emotional high, a painful dose of reality wallops me in the face. None was more painful than the phone call we received in the middle of the night. My daughter Kathi had just had an emergency C-section to deliver her triplets, who weren't due until July.

Although the triplets were more than three months premature, and therefore very, very small, at first they seemed to be doing well. By the time Gerri and I got back to San Diego, that had all changed. The smallest boy, Tyler, and the little girl, Jordyn, suffered massive bleeding in both hemispheres of the brain, while Dylan had less extensive bleeding on one side of the brain. Within a week, we had lost two of the children and knew that Dylan would face some serious problems.

I think I speak for most parents and grandparents when I say that if I could have traded my life for theirs, I would have done it in a heartbeat. Fighting for my own survival had become second nature to me. But in this circumstance I was lost. It seemed so unfair. I had already led a wonderful life; I had done, seen, and accomplished so much and these tiny little babies hadn't had a chance for any life at all. Losing them, and watching the pain that my daughter was going through, with absolutely no way to help or change any of it, was one of the most painful things I have ever experienced. Over the past nine years, I have watched Dylan go through more medical procedures and deal with more problems than most adults ever do. Yet he maintains the sunniest disposition and leads a happy and full life. I can't tell you the joy it brings me to watch him get out on the field and give it all he has to kick a soccer ball, or hit a baseball. Life will not be easy for him, and my hope is that I can be around for a long time to help him as much as possible.

Gerri

The high we experienced after the success of the vaccine was undeniable, but it was followed by very low lows. First, there was Kathi's terrible loss, and then there were more mysterious seizures.

In September of 1999, Brian came out of the shower, got dressed, and told me that he was taking Steve for a ride out on the boat.

This would have seemed like a fine idea except for the fact that we were in Ireland, Steve was in San Diego, and we didn't have a boat.

Brian seemed annoyed when I tried to point this out to him, and assuming the self-assured attitude of a trial attorney, he made it seem as if I must be the one who was mixed up. I literally had to push him down onto the bed and hold on to him so he wouldn't leave the room. Within a few minutes, he was back to normal, but I was at a loss. All scans had showed the tumors were gone. What exactly was going on?

The first round of the vaccine program was over and we had rewarded ourselves with a trip to Ireland. My son Todd and his wife, Jennifer, joined us. Todd is an avid golfer and was looking forward to playing on some of Ireland's amazing courses, and Jennifer welcomed the chance to get away. I must admit that I had an ulterior motive in asking them along, though—I didn't want to go on this trip without help. Brian had started to have problems with reading. He could work his way through any text, but where he once could just breeze along, now he labored over it. Dr. McDermott had told me that it was likely the result of some radiation damage. The problem was fairly minor at this point, but Todd had noticed and, fabulous son that he is, worked out a plan so Brian never knew anything was amiss.

Brian had decided that Todd would be the designated driver throughout the trip, something Todd was more than happy to handle. Brian was navigator, but it quickly became obvious to the rest of us that Brian could not decipher the road signs and the map quickly enough to really navigate. He had been through so much, and it would have added insult to injury to "demote" him now. So every night Todd took the map to his room and memorized the route for the next day. When Brian couldn't give the directions in time, Todd would say something about having just noticed a sign that made him think we should make this particular turn right, and what did Brian think? Brian was happy to take Todd's recommendations and the trip went along without incident.

But the boat conversation was alarming. A concerned phone call to Mike McDermott gave me the explanation that Brian had suffered a small focal seizure. He said that this is pretty common after neurosurgery, and was likely a result of the buildup of scar tissue over the site where the tumor had been removed during the craniotomy. Todd was the one who came up with the best nonmedical explanation of it. He described it as a record that has a piece of dust on it. Most of the time when the needle encounters the dust, it simply goes over it, but every once in a while, the needle gets stuck. As long as the needle didn't get stuck too often, we were okay. Unfortunately, Brian's needle began to get stuck more and more frequently.

As soon as we returned from Ireland, Dr. McDermott ordered another MRI and the great news was that everything looked all clear once again. McDermott said that as long as there were good intervals between these episodes and Brian's motor functions weren't involved, the problem was acceptable.

"Acceptable" was a good word. As long as I knew that what was happening to Brian wasn't life-threatening, I decided that I would just have to deal with it.

Still, while I understood the problem on an intellectual level, it felt like a punch in the stomach every time Brian's "needle" got stuck. And these moments always came out of the blue. Within a minute, I could go from having a normal conversation with my husband to facing a person who recognized me but couldn't say my name. Brian came out of each of these episodes totally exhausted, and I did, too. It wasn't easy, but there wasn't a choice: we simply had to handle it as best we could.

At one point I told Dr. McDermott that I didn't remember his ever mentioning this kind of damage as a possibility. With a small, wry smile, he replied, "I'm not sure that we expected Brian to live this long. He's beaten all the odds."

From a medical standpoint, the doctors had realized that such a problem could arise, but their main focus had been on Brian's survival. And even if we had understood that the Gamma Knife surgery and craniotomy might result in these word problems and the aphasia that followed, we would have followed the same course of action. As I often tell Brian, "There is no free lunch."

Brian

Throughout the next eleven months, I continued to have small, intermittent focal seizures. But the time lapse between them began to shorten and by midsummer of 2000, we were back in San Francisco for more CT scans and MRIs to find out whether more surgery was necessary. Thankfully, no evidence of any tumor activity had shown up on previous scans; but there was a definite possibility of my needing surgery to remove or shave down the scar tissue on the surface of my brain that was causing the seizures. A few days later, Mike McDermott called with the test results.

"I have good news and bad news," he said. This time, I took the bad news first. "The bad news is that you have to have a second craniotomy. The good news is that you won't have to be awake during it."

The not being awake part was good. But when I passed the phone to Gerri, I simply and quietly said, "Shit." I was not expressive, not crying, not angry, but a wave of depression swept over me.

Our dog, Joy, had been with us for a year and a half, and up to that moment it was clear that she was more Gerri's dog than mine. When the phone rang, she had been sitting by Gerri's side. But when I reacted to the news from Dr. McDermott, Joy did something she had never done before. She moved over to me, leaned against me, put her black Labrador face on my lap, and looked up at me with a look that clearly said, "I'm sorry, buddy. I'm here for you."

Instinctively, she had known that I needed her. From that moment on, she became my dog.

Let me explain. For several years prior to my diagnosis, Gerri had been pushing for us to get a dog. While we both loved them, I had fought back against this idea with the hard-headed, realistic argument that with work or travel, we were both gone too much and it simply wouldn't be fair to the animal. Thankfully, Gerri didn't give up. She had learned about Canine Companions, a nonprofit organization that enhances the lives of disabled individuals by providing them with very special, highly trained assistance dogs. But the dogs who "flunk out" of the program are pretty special, too. Intelligent, loyal, and housebroken, they can respond to about two pages of commands. About six months after my diagnosis, we had received a call saying that one of these dogs was available. We were told that although she was one of the best dogs they had ever had, she had one problem: she was "ball intensive." That meant that while she might be the best trained dog in the world, pulling a wheelchair along with all her might, if a tennis ball rolled by there was no doubt she'd go right after it. The poor person in the wheelchair would be history!

Since we thought that the vaccine therapy was about to start, I didn't believe the timing was great. But I knew that Gerri had been operating under incredible stress on my behalf, and I thought that having a dog would be good for her. So Joy came into our lives. In both body and spirit.

Intelligent as she is, Joy probably understood that I had been against this whole dog idea at first, but her special training and sensitivity to patients in need led her to come to my side when I needed her most. And believe me, she hasn't left it since. Throughout this struggle, Joy has given me all the love, affection, and enduring acceptance a dog can give. At times she's been the best therapy in the world.

Get a Dog

Advocate Tip #39

Brian and I have since learned about studies suggesting that some dogs seem to have the ability to sense the existence of cancer and other diseases. Even if that were not the case, it is very clear that these animals bring a wonderful tranquillity to our lives. Dogs are being brought into nursing homes and hospitals because their very presence is consoling; they calm patients and speed up the healing process. I believe that if you and/or your patient are in a position to have such a faithful companion, your patient's journey through medical treatments can only be made easier by it. If you and your patient can't own a dog, try to spend time with someone who has a pet. Form a bond with it. For more information on getting a pet specially trained to aid people facing disease, see page 213.

Dr. McDermott went on to describe this second surgery to us as pretty simple and straightforward. Finally reassured, I began to tell everyone that it was going to be a "no-brainer."

Although the thought of brain surgery is always intimidating, I approached this second craniotomy with a weird sense of relief. I was just so damned happy I didn't have to be awake while they worked inside my skull. After the first craniotomy, I had made a vow that I would never submit to another one. But maybe it's like childbirth. As long as there's something good that comes out of it, you forget about how difficult it was to go through the first time. I knew I would be in the hands of the best medical team possible, and I concentrated on focusing on the upside.

Just before the surgery, on August 24th, Dr. McDermott came in to the pre-op room and asked whether I had any questions. "After this surgery, will I be able to play the piano?"

Mike looked at me quizzically. "I expect so."

"That's great. I've never been able to do it before."

It's an old joke, and I should have been ashamed of myself for telling it, but then again I have no shame. Susan and Steve Parker were once again with us for the surgery. Besides providing moral support and comfort, they always laugh at my jokes. At least Susan does.

A few minutes later, the anesthesiologist arrived to go over his role in the surgery. He was young, standing about 6 feet 4 and weighing in at about 200 pounds, obviously in good shape. Gerri looked up at him and asked, "Did they bring you in to make sure Brian doesn't try to escape again?" He laughed and said, "I've heard talk."

The surgery was uneventful. Since I was knocked out and made no attempts to climb off the table or stop the proceedings, it was probably pretty boring for Mike McDermott and the rest of the crew.*

*For Dr. Mike McDermott's perspective on why Brian's outcome has been successful, see page 210.

Gerri

The morning after the second craniotomy, I showed up at the hospital with a deck of playing cards. Brian's head was swathed in bandages, his arms still hooked up to IVs. The nurse in the ICU looked at me, aghast, as I dealt my husband a gin rummy hand. "Oh, sweetie, I really don't think your husband is up to playing cards this morning," she said.

"That's what I'm hoping for," I told her. I was determined to at least walk away from this ordeal with one win against the man who never loses, even at cards. Brian understood exactly what I was trying to do, and he stopped laughing long enough to win, as always. Do you have any idea of the damage that has been done to my pride by losing at gin rummy to a guy with brain tumors?

Treat Doctors, Nurses, and Medical Staff Well

Brian and I always tried to make the medical professionals see us as individuals rather than "the patient in 207." When speaking with them, we always worked in stories about our grandchildren, or the local baseball team, or something other than Brian's medical condition. When they came rushing into the exam room, I found that I could always slow them down a little bit by saying, "It looks as if you're having a tough day. What's going on?" Asking them how they were doing before we ever started to talk about Brian often broke the ice. Also, I really don't think whining ever works, so we tried to deal with doctors and nurses in a positive tone. Doctors always chuckled when they asked Brian how he was doing and his response was, "I'm great. Except for this cancer thing. So let's get rid of that."

Brian is such an outgoing guy that it's his nature to reach out and shake hands with everyone he meets. I've often laughed at the startled looks on the faces of the nurses' assistants or janitors or physical therapists when they came into his room and Brian would reach out his hand and say, "Hi, I'm Brian. What's your name?" By the time they left the room he had made a new friend, and I have to believe that if they could, they would go the extra mile for him.

My personality is not nearly as outgoing as Brian's. But I could, and did, let everyone from the receptionists to the neurosurgeons know that we appreciated what they were trying to do for him. I knew that they all had bad days and bad situations to deal with, and I expressed my understanding of that. It was easy for me to say to a nurse in ICU, "I know that I'm not supposed to be here, but I promise I'll stay out of your way. I know you're swamped and have way too much to do. If you need me out of here, just tell me. But please let me just sit here quietly and let Brian know that I'm here for him."

In this cost-cutting medical world, the nurses—especially the nurses—know that their patient contact time is too often limited. I've had nurses and doctors tell me that if they have a loved one in the hospital, they want to be there with that patient on a constant basis. Over and over again, I had nurses tell me that in my position, they would be doing the exact same thing I was doing: being an advocate for my husband, questioning the medicine they were giving him, asking them for advice, being there as much as possible.

Another way to interact on a human level and thus get the best care for your patient is to offer to help overworked medical staff. If they said Brian could have fruit juice, I offered to run to the refrigerator to get it. Usually they said no, but that offer let them know I was willing to do anything, be the gofer, do any errand that needed to be done, and that above all, I wasn't expecting them to wait on us or trying to cause any extra work for them. Cookies, candy, or doughnuts always helped. Seriously. You don't have to make a big deal of it. Just put the treat on the counter at the nurses' station. They always figure it out.

Brian

My recovery from this second operation was very easy. We stayed in San Francisco for a few days before returning to San Diego. During this time, Gerri and I were once again blown away by the fact that only in San Francisco can you go into a nice restaurant with your head swathed in bandages and have not one person so much as glance at you. Anyhow, this time they had shaved most of my head and the hair began to grow back quickly into its normal thick thatch. I'm lucky that way. If I were bald, I'd be one really ugly guy with all those cuts, bumps, and grooves. Gerri says that the scars made my head look like a baseball. Fortunately, I'm a living Chia Pet!

Everything had gone so smoothly that once again I was lulled into thinking that the crisis was over for good. What a blockhead! Some people just don't get the picture!

Back in January of 2000, when the millennium was celebrated, I was more than ready to turn the page. In my usual (some would say, overly) optimistic approach, I felt that I was now "over cancer" and my life could move forward in a new direction. It had been a tough eighteen months, with the Gamma Knife, a lymphadenectomy, an open craniotomy, and the experimental dendritic-cell program. But my last MRIs and CT scans had been clean. It was over. We had won!

I was ready to focus on a new path, a new "mission" in life. I knew that it wasn't possible for me to keep practicing law. It was time for me to re-create myself as a person: if I couldn't be a lawyer, I decided that I would channel my passion into other efforts.

I sent a letter to friends, clients, and colleagues telling them that I was shutting down my life's work, my law practice of thirty years. First, I thanked the attorneys who had mentored me along the way. I expressed my gratitude for all the help I had received from clients, fellow lawyers and judges, The Lads, my children, and Gerri. The letter was filled with hope and optimism and plans for the future.

I spoke of serving on several boards: the American Ireland Fund, Hastings College of the Law, and the San Diego Padres. I also wanted to pay back those mentors from thirty years ago by doing the same thing for young lawyers preparing to do trial work. I indicated that I had plans to spend time as a volunteer judge in Judge Jim Milliken's invigorated juvenile court system, helping to turn the lives of young offenders around. So my plans were laid. I was no longer a trial lawyer but I was prepared to do good, in my own way to pay it forward.

I didn't expect much in the way of responses, but as the days passed, a torrent reached my office. They were wonderful letters, and if I had any lingering thoughts of feeling sorry for myself, they took care of that. My favorite was from Dr. Richard Braun, a hand surgeon and former client who said, "Brian, the Holy Bench has given you a wonderful continuance."

True, but have you ever heard the Jewish proverb that says, "Man plans. God laughs"?

I think God must like to laugh as much as I do. He sure as hell has laughed at a lot of the plans I've made!

Chapter Nine

MAKE YOUR LIFE WORTH LIVING

Whether you think you can or think you can't, you're right.
—HENRY FORD

Brian

In September 2000, three weeks after my second craniotomy, I sat down in my favorite chair, turned on the TV, and began watching the Summer Olympics. Then suddenly, nothing worked. I felt as if a deep fog had settled over me and I just sat there in a kind of stupor. It was as if I had become frozen in time.

At that moment, my war went from a battle against cancer to the most enduring, most profound, and in my view, most challenging medical crisis: a long-term battle against aphasia. I went straight from the fight for my life into a fight to make my life worth living.

Aphasia. Technically, I think they label it as a disorder that results from damage to the language center of the brain. How nice. In reality, it's the bottom of the barrel. The pits. It affects your ability to speak, to comprehend, and often, the ability to read and write. While stroke is the most common cause of aphasia, it can also be caused by traumatic brain injury. The numbers tell us that approximately one million individuals in the United States have aphasia, and it is estimated that 80,000 people are afflicted each year. That's a lot of people in the same boat. The everyday struggle faced by stroke victims is the same drawn-out battle faced by a young college kid who suffers a traumatic brain injury in a car accident, a young soldier returning from war with a closed head injury, or a sixty-year-old trial attorney who made his living by speaking to juries, who was now struggling for every word.

Is that you laughing again, God?

Gerri

I had left Brian alone for just a short time while I went to the grocery store. When I returned, he was sitting in front of the television and didn't turn to greet me. This was the first sign that something was wrong. I walked over to his chair only to find him staring straight ahead, blankly, at the screen.

"Brian, are you all right?" I demanded.

His only reply was a strange grunt. I noticed that his sandwich was half-eaten and his Coke still had ice cubes in it. Whatever was going on with him must have just happened. It was clear that he was unable to talk. I dumped the groceries on the counter and called Dan Einhorn, the very same friend who had given us Brian's diagnosis back in May of 1998. Dan dropped everything and met us at the hospital. He contacted Mike McDermott in San Francisco and together they arranged for an MRI and other tests, and also brought in a neurologist to quarterback the team.

While the doctors were performing all these tests in an effort to find out what was going on, Brian was a complete mess. He couldn't do anything. He couldn't tell anyone his name. He literally couldn't say one word that was intelligible, and unlike the problems he had in the past, this didn't go away. For the next few days, Brian was unable to do anything for himself. I had to "teach" him how to get into a car, folding up his legs for him and putting them inside. He couldn't go to the bathroom by himself. He couldn't hold a fork, feed himself, or dress himself. This vigorous hunk of a man sat in front of me as helpless as an infant. His response to any question was complete nonsense. By the second day, when a nurse asked him his name, he replied, "Kiss, Kiss, Kiss." Sweet words in one sense, yet terrifying for me. There was nothing I could do, and all my efforts at being an advocate seemed to have led us nowhere.

Facing down cancer and brain tumors was not nearly as terrible as this. This was the one time that I didn't think in terms of the word "hope." For a while, there didn't seem to be any. As for Brian, it was the first time that he was truly frustrated. I had seen him go through major surgeries with nary a whimper, but during the first few days of his hospitalization after the major seizure, tears of frustration streamed down his face. Brian, who loves being around people and is really energized by them, didn't want to see anyone. Or rather, he didn't want anyone to see him the way he was. At first, he only allowed his good friend Steve Parker to visit. Over the next few days he allowed a few more people to come, but this time there were no parties, no napkins and cutlery, and no laughter.

It was incredibly frustrating for me to be unable to help him. I'm a doer, and now I could do nothing. As I sat in the hospital room that first day or so, and saw Brian completely unable to do anything for himself, I began planning our new life. I made the decision that if he remained in this state, Brian would not go into a nursing home, but that we would turn our home office/ guest room into a residence for a caregiver. I started calculating the savings we had and decided that I would just exhaust them if I needed to. I knew immediately that I would be unable to care for Brian by myself on a 24/7 basis, as there is simply no way I could move my big guy around.

In short, I felt I was facing something I wouldn't be able to handle. I can go toe to toe with just about anyone, but looking into the eyes of the person I loved and seeing total fear, panic, frustration, and confusion was enough to leave me wanting to curl up into a tight little ball and go to sleep.

Just when I was feeling my lowest, I experienced a moment that helped me to remember something every advocate needs to know: that just by being there, hour after hour, involved as Brian's advocate, I was doing something. One night, as I stood by the nurses station after an endless day spent by Brian's side, one of the nurses began to chat.

"You two have been married a long time, haven't you?"

"What makes you say that?"

"Well, we sit here and see what's going on with our patients. With our years of practice, we've learned that we can pick out the couples who've been married for a long time, because that spouse is always here for the other one. If they haven't been married very long, the other person often begins to feel that this life, with all the trauma that's going on, isn't what they signed on for. And they begin to fall away. They just don't show up much. We've watched you, and you're here all day, every day, and you're going to be a major part of your husband's recovery. So tell me. How long have you been married?"

"Five years."

The nurse paused for a moment, leaned her head to one side and gave me a little smile. She reached out and patted my arm. "Good for you. Your husband is a lucky guy." It remains one of my proudest moments. All too often, it's easy to overlook the toll that a major illness takes on the caregiver, the advocate. We naturally focus our attention and concern on the patient, and the advocate usually gets short shrift. One of the major lessons I've learned from this experience is that we need to help the helper.

Get Others to Help

Advocate Tip
#41

One of the best ways to help an advocate is to validate the worth of the effort being put forth, just as the nurse did for me. That exhausted person plunked down next to the bedside needs affirmation from others that he or she is indeed making a difference.

Speaking from experience, I can tell you that it's often difficult for the advocate to accept help. Once you become an advocate, it becomes easy to fall into a pattern of thinking that asking for help is a sign of weakness or a shirking of duty. So if you know people going through a tough, drawn-out medical crisis, you need to step in with specific offers of help. Don't just say, "Please let us know if there's anything we can do to help." That's too general. Instead, ask, "Can I take your dog for a walk? Can I pick up some groceries for you? Can I drive your patient to the doctor's next Wednesday? Can I spend some time with him while you go to work out? When are you getting your hair done? Can I come by and spend some time with your patient then? Would it be okay if I come over sometime next Tuesday and have coffee with him while you go hit a bucket of balls? What time works best for you?" The more specific the date, the time, and the offer of help, the more likely it is that it will be accepted.

Drop by the hospital for a quick visit. And don't go empty-handed. Bring a few bottles of water (hospitals are notoriously "arid"), which will likely be consumed, and greatly appreciated, by the advocate if not the patient. Bring a piece of fruit or two, but don't forget a napkin or even better, some of those wet wipes. Homemade baked goods are always appreciated. I bake a mean pumpkin bread and always bring one to patients and their advocates in the hospital. It's extra thoughtful if you slice it beforehand!

There are many things you can do that can give a patient and advocate the feeling of being enveloped in a warm hug. When we began this fight in May of 1998, we were ready to head out the door for a month-long trip to Italy. That didn't happen. But a week or so after we canceled that trip and were on our rounds to doctor after doctor, we arrived home totally exhausted one evening to find a basket on our doorstep. It contained a jar of pasta sauce, some pasta, a bottle of Italian wine, and a CD of Italian songs by Andrea Boccelli. The note from Susan and Craig McClellan read, "We know that you couldn't go to Italy, so we thought we would bring a slice of Italy to you. We love you and are thinking about you." That simple gesture warmed our hearts. Indeed, we've duplicated that gesture with other friends who are going through difficult times, and it always gets the same response we had felt.

Neighbors or friends can organize a dinner club. It takes someone who is willing to take charge, but it's not that difficult to do. Start with your e-mail list and look for friends you have in common. Send an e-mail asking them if they would like to help the Smiths by bringing them dinner one night every other week for the next month. Which night would be best for them? What would they like to make for dinner? It doesn't have to be a meal for every night of the week, but even a few can help take some of the strain off. Not having to prepare a meal when you are inundated with medical problems can be a great gift.

When a medical crisis finally gets to the stage of being a long, protracted battle, allowing the advocate to get away for a few days is a huge boost in the recovery process for both the advocate and, by extension, the patient. Getting relief from the feeling of being completely tied down was wonderful for me, especially after our grandchildren began arriving and I had my "Nana" urge to go see them. Because it will be so difficult for the advocate to believe he or she can break away without causing harm to the patient, it's likely that it will take a family member or very close friend to step in and make this offer of assistance. The Parkers are such good friends and care about Brian so much that I was truly comfortable in leaving him with them for a few days. They couldn't have given me a better gift.

For more resources on how to help friends who are going through a medical crisis and need more long-term care, see page 213.

Brian

I need to jump in here. I think it's incredibly important for patients, too, to realize that they need to take some responsibility for the care of their advocates. Your advocate is working like hell to save your life, and there are a few little things that you can do that would be appreciated.

Sending flowers is one of them. Even if you're stuck in the hospital, a quick call to a florist can brighten the advocate's day. (That's if you can figure out how to dial an outside line!) I'm one of those guys who has a hard and fast rule against what I call Hallmark holidays. If I'm told that I should send flowers, I don't. But when I was really sick and didn't have the strength to do much else, I did find a nurse to help me order flowers for Gerri. Her reaction when the nurse walked in carrying a vase filled with a dozen long-stemmed red roses and, wearing a big smile, handed them to her, not me, was worth the effort.

When someone asks you, the patient, if there's anything they can do to help, tell them, "You bet." Ask them to stay with you while your advocate gets a chance to go exercise or see a movie, or go out to lunch. Gerri can demand the moon and the stars for me, but she really has trouble asking for help for herself. It was far better for me to let others know that she could use some relief. I felt that by doing the asking, I was able to help her. It was a win-win situation for each of us!

Gerri

While we were waiting to hear test results, I felt completely drained and exhausted. It took everything I had to maintain some outward sign of cheerfulness and hope when I was around Brian. There were times when I took a break from his bedside and walked up and down the parking lot of the hospital, tears pouring down my face. I even had conversations with myself.

"I don't think I can do this."

"Yes, you can. What are the alternatives?"

Advocate Tip
#42

Take Care of Yourself

Someone needs to be looking out for the advocate, and while others can help, the person who can do that best is you. Hopefully, you'll be blessed with friends and family who are willing to spell you whenever they can. But by and large, you will be the laboring oar. So it's up to you to do whatever it takes to keep yourself healthy. If you can get a massage every so often, do it. If you can break away and go to a movie, do it. Take some time out to do whatever makes you feel good. Of paramount importance is taking the time to exercise. Get the endorphins working for you. If you spend an hour walking or running or doing aerobics a few times a week, you will not be wasting time on yourself. And you'll make up for any "wasted" hours by being more productive and able to focus and think more clearly. In effect, by taking care of yourself, you can take better care of your patient.

Brian

My inability to function went on for three days until the diagnosis of post-surgical seizures explained the situation. I was given a drug called Dilantin to control the unremitting seizure activity in my brain, and within a few hours I had significant improvement. I slowly began to regain my motor functions, but my thought processes remained out of whack.

I was enough aware of what was going on to feel total confusion and frustration, which over the next day or so evolved into anger. Dr. Rolf Ehlers, an internist with a great reputation, was brought in to help manage my case, but I absolutely refused to talk to him or make any attempt to answer his questions. Dr. Ehlers has a strong German accent, which must have reminded me of Sigmund Freud, because in my confusion, I decided that Ehlers was a shrink. I was angry that anyone could possibly think I was "wacko." Dr. Ehlers has now become my personal physician and I consider him a friend, but at that moment, I wanted to have nothing to do with him. I definitely had periods of strong paranoia. At one point, I was convinced that the air ducts in the ceiling contained people who were spying on me. Nothing Gerri said or did could change my mind. Even a few days later, when I was able to walk around, I believed that I could hear all the other patients whispering about me. I kept turning to Gerri and saying, "Do you hear that? They're all talking about me! Do you hear them?" The irony was that I had spent much of my life hoping that people were talking about me, and now I was afraid of it!

One day, my daughter, Kathi, brought our then seventeen-month-old grandson, Dylan, into my hospital room. Dylan had suffered tremendously as a result of his premature birth and mild case of cerebral palsy. While I recognized that Kathi and Dylan were standing before me, I was unable to even recall their names. I knew who they were, but terrifyingly, I couldn't remember the name of my own daughter. Kathi placed Dylan at the foot of my bed and, with no prompting, he crawled all the way up until he reached my face and hugged my neck. Although I'm not sure I could fully comprehend it at that time, I somehow understood that we were fighting the same sort of battle—our bodies were just not doing what they were supposed to do. I broke into tears.

Gerri had been by my side on an almost constant basis throughout this hospitalization, and now that I've learned the importance of a great advocate, I really understand how important her presence was. By about 11:00 p.m. on the third evening, when she could see that the Dilantin was starting to take effect, she finally went home, totally exhausted.

I might have been unintelligible but that didn't mean that I couldn't think, and right then, with Gerri gone, I focused on one thought: "ESCAPE." I had one of those "Brian Monaghan moments." I'd had enough, and more than anything I wanted out of that hospital. Right then. I was stuck there with no money, no car, and no clothing other than that joke of a nightgown they give you (and at 6 feet 3, the joke was on me). I knew that Gerri wouldn't help me to escape, but there was one person I knew I could depend on, my good friend of so many years, Steve Parker. I knew that if I called Parker, he would come get me, and so I picked up the phone next to my bed and over and over I tried to dial an outside line. With each of my attempts, the nurse came into my room. At first with disdain, and eventually disgust, I waved the nurse away. Over and over again I repeated this. It wasn't until the next day that I learned that the phone I was using to get an outside line was nothing more than the nurses' call button, which I was frantically pushing again and again. Since I was in the neurosurgery ward, hospital rules dictated that the nurses could not simply ignore the call button. After an hour or so of my placing "calls," the nurses decided that the only way to calm me down was to get Gerri. So at one o'clock in the morning, they called her at home and asked for her help in dealing with me.

Within a short time Gerri was back at the hospital, and while she was exhausted, she was also incredibly happy. We now knew that focal seizures resulting from my surgeries were causing my problem. The Dilantin had really begun to take effect, and the brain seizures were beginning to come under control. While I had been completely focused on the possibility of escaping my prison cell, I had not even noticed that I was now able to speak—coherently. Apparently, I was not overly excited by this fantastic development. I was still focused on escape. Gerri, however, was ecstatic and kept saying, "Brian, you're talking. You can talk!"

Instead of recognizing the importance of this huge step forward and rejoicing in it, I kept muttering, "Parker would have gotten me out of here." Finally, in order to prevent a possible escape, Gerri crawled into the hospital bed with me. She draped her body half over mine and soon fell into an exhausted sleep. I didn't get back to sleep for a long time, but I remember that I stayed as quiet as I could so as not to waken her.

When I left the hospital a week later, I knew that I was one of the lucky ones. All of my motor functions had returned to normal and I was able to take care of myself. In a sense. I learned that these activities are called ADLs, or activities of daily living. They are the things we all take for granted every day, all day. But when they are taken from you, even for a short time, you realize that the simple act of brushing your teeth is a blessing. You know that being able to dress yourself or take care of your bathroom needs are things we learned as kids, and no adult wants to be treated as a child. So I was lucky to leave the hospital with my motor functions intact. But "lucky" doesn't really describe what I felt. Profoundly grateful is more like it.

Although I could take care of my daily needs, there's no doubt that my life was still severely affected. To the casual observer I seemed normal. But although I could speak pretty coherently, I was unable to decode words from individual letters. The only way that I can describe my inability to read is to say that it was almost as though I had been picked up in the middle of the night and dropped off on a city street in China or Afghanistan. The advertisements, directions, and signs were incomprehensible to me. I was able to recognize the letters themselves, I just didn't understand their meaning. And I couldn't access words in speech when I needed to, either. Unlike when I was recovering from the brain surgery itself, when my half-shaved head or surgery scars were outside and visible, all of the problems were now *inside* my head.

To me it seemed as though God was saying "Okay, Brian, I am making you an offer. You can live. You will be allowed to spend time with Gerri and you will get to enjoy your grandchildren. You will be able to be with your children, your friends, and loved ones. But there will be a cost for these gifts. You will not be able to read. You will no longer be able to give lectures or speeches. You will have to give up your plans to volunteer as a juvenile court judge. And you must spend time giving back to others. Is that a deal, Brian?" That would be a classic "offer you can't refuse"!

Gerri

Within a day of Brian's getting home, I knew that we needed to find a quality speech therapist for him. Once again, I asked friends for help in finding the best and was given the name of Diane Johnson. When I checked with our health insurance company, I found that insurance would only pay for Brian to take part in "group" speech therapy sessions. I asked for more details and learned that the "group" could consist of people suffering from very severe, long-term aphasia, as well as people like Brian who weren't as severely affected. It was easy to see that Brian was going through lots of frustration, and even depression. I knew that he would need to see some quick progress in his recovery or it would be too easy to give up. I made another one of what Brian calls my executive decisions, and signed us up for private sessions with the speech therapist of our choice.

Advocate Tip #43

Get Private or Semi-Private Therapy

This is something that is vitally important to enable a patient to recover to the fullest extent possible. Once again we were lucky in that we were able to pay for private speech therapy sessions when our insurance wouldn't cover them. If you have the financial means, now is a time when it's worth opening your wallet to pay for this on your own. If you need to swallow your pride and put out the word to take up a collection, or borrow money from a friend, this is when you simply must do it. We're talking about therapy that will affect your loved one every day for the rest of his or her life—and your life as well. Both Brian and I have come to believe so strongly in this that, if it becomes necessary for you to refinance your home to pay for private therapy, we would recommend that you do it. Getting individualized help, often and early, is crucial.

Brian

In dealing with my aphasia, just as I had with the cancer itself, I once again decided to "write the ending first." I set myself three main goals, which boiled down to: 1) learn to speak fluently; 2) learn to read; and 3) regain my sense of independence. I decided that all I had to do to achieve the third objective was to accomplish the first two. Then I looked at what tools I needed in order to get to the finish line. All three of those new tasks required the same 'tude I had brought to the fight in dealing with cancer. I decided that I didn't care what I had to do, what hell I had to go through, what miserable frustration I had to overcome in getting to the point where I was once again "literate." But this time, I had to accomplish most of this on my own. Gerri could and did point me in the right direction, hooking me up with my wonderful speech therapist Diane Johnson, but there wasn't much else she could do for my recovery itself. This time, it was up to me. With that knowledge came a greater sense of stick-to-itiveness. It was as though my mom was once again demanding that I "go back there and hit him again, right in the nose" or my old football coach was saying "we're going to do it again, till we get it right."

Like most aphasia victims, I often have problems finding the word I want to say. As I'm about to speak a particular word, it just disappears. I can't get hold of it. Too often, I seem fixated on a word that I totally understand in my head, but I can't find, or say, the word. My speech therapist has spent hours helping me with a technique that allows me not to keep butting up against a brick wall, trying over and over to say the same word, but instead to sort of slide off to find another word that will describe what I'm trying to say. One time I turned to Gerri and said "1-2-2-5. The guy with the white beard." It helps to be married to an "Irish witch" who can read my mind, but when you think about it, that was a pretty logical way to say the word "Christmas."

Of the three major goals, the most significant facet of aphasia for me was (and is) the inability to read normally. I have spent hours every day, every week of the last eight years working on

153

getting back my ability to read. And while I can now read, it's slow. Damned slow. To those who can read, this problem is hard to comprehend. But just think about it. Reading is everywhere. You go check into a doctor's office, and they hand you a form to fill out. You take your car in for some work, and they hand you a form to fill out. You go to check into a hotel, same story. Take a look at a menu: it's written! Try to get away from it all by going to a movie. Until you can't read, you don't appreciate how often movies flash a written word across the screen to indicate a time or place, like "Moscow, 1999." And everything is flashed at you so quickly. Sometimes I want to yell out, "Hey! Leave it up there for a while. I can read the damn thing if you'll just give me a chance!"

Eight years later, it takes me days (yes, days!) just to write one page of the book you are holding in your hands. And then Gerri has to help rework it. Because although the concept of what I want to say is clearly in my mind, as I sit down to write something it seems to take forever for me to be able to translate those thoughts onto the page.

Whether it's fighting cancer, or aphasia, or even playing sports, there is a need to psych yourself up to achieve your objective. Watch a professional football player getting ready to start a game. He has been playing his sport through grammar school, high school, college, and now the NFL. He knows what he needs to do. Why does he jump up and down, yelling and beating his teammates on the top of the head? To reach the highest level of performance requires focused mental concentration and physical intensity. It's not just sports. As a lawyer, I had tried more than a hundred jury trials and knew what I needed to do. Yet as you'll recall, the night before each trial I would replay that *Patton* speech, and we headed off to court the following morning listening to the theme song from *Rocky*. It may seem silly, but it's a question of psyching yourself up to reach your highest level. Or at times, psyching yourself up just to get out of bed.

There is no denying the fact that it's tough to hype yourself each day. The first part of the battle is often the easiest; initially, it's easy to think that you will, once again, overcome all odds and walk away from this problem a winner. At least, that's how

154

it was for me. At first I was in the absolute depths of frustration. When, a few days later, I regained the ability to eat, drink, talk, and be merry, I was once again a happy and grateful camper. Then came the reality that aphasia and its accompanying problems had changed my life forever. Fighting a battle against cancer was easier for me than facing the fact that my life would never be the same again. I had to pick myself up, psych myself into moving forward, one step—or in my case, one word—at a time.

Gather Inspirational Stories

Advocate Tip #44

If you haven't realized it by now, Brian and I are firm believers in the power of stories to inspire hope. One of the things that helped Brian most during his long-term battle against aphasia was to read (okay, listen to is more like it!) some extraordinary books, stories of people who had used every ounce of their being to fortify themselves, to keep putting one foot in front of the other, until they got where they needed to be. Whether it's an amazing tale of an underdog racehorse or the story of an explorer's arctic adventure, stories can inspire your patient, too. For a list of some of Brian's favorites, see page 216.

If your patient isn't much of a book person, rent some movies that will inspire. It may sound obvious, but I'd recommend steering away from tearjerkers about death and dying. When in doubt, remember that laughter can be the best medicine of all, so bring them comedies you know will tickle their funny bone. Whether it's the Three Stooges or Will Farrell, giving your patient something to laugh about may inspire a new and happier outlook.

Gerri

Of all the terrible things that Brian has gone through, it's the lonely, quiet battle he has waged against aphasia that has made me the proudest. We all take reading for granted, and so did Brian until he had to relearn the alphabet. Actually, it was more frustrating than learning to read in the first place, since the pride he took in reading a particular word one minute could be wiped out ten minutes later when he couldn't recognize the same word. The frustration level from this aspect alone was huge; it wasn't as though he could "learn" the word if he just tried hard enough. His brain already knew the word, but sometimes refused to recognize it. The analogy his speech therapist used was that it was as if someone had rearranged everything in all the cabinets and closets in his house. Everything is still there, but it takes a long time to find them.

I feel certain that if I were faced with aphasia, I'd have withdrawn from the world and hidden in my cave. Not only did Brian refuse to hide, he was willing to reach out for whatever help he could get to overcome this problem. On Christmas 2000, our grandson Riley Wortmann, fifteen months at the time, received an electronic toy used to learn the alphabet. When asked to find a particular letter, if the correct button was pressed, an obnoxious, penetrating voice would announce the letter and then say, "Good job!" If the wrong button was pressed, a buzzer went off and the voice said, "Try again." Brian took one look at the toy and said, "Riley's too young for this. I'd like to borrow it." No one has ever accused Brian Monaghan of not having an ego, but he rose above any shame he felt at using a child's toy to help him relearn the alphabet, so determined was he to overcome his loss.

Brian's progress has been amazing. A few years ago, his speech therapist told Brian that in all the time she had worked with patients with aphasia, she'd never seen anyone overcome it as well as he had. She said that his ability was truly unique and—very seriously—asked him if he would consider donating his brain to science so researchers could try to determine what set him apart from other patients. When Brian came home with this news, he found me sitting at the kitchen table, stacks of paperwork spread out before me, working my way through the medical bills—never a good time for me. With great (and justifiable) pride, Brian told me that Diane wanted him to donate his brain to science. Apparently, I wasn't having my best day, because I looked up at him and snapped, "Is she willing to wait awhile or does she want it right now?"

Brian's spirit through all of this has been magnificent, and (my sarcasm in this instance aside) I am in awe of it. He has continued to work on his aphasia ceaselessly. One of the things that has given him much comfort is that there have been many times when we've met new people who never realize that Brian has a problem at all. Or, as he says, they just think he has "old-timer's," like everyone else his age.

Once life got back to "normal," or what had become our new normal, I recognized that I would wear myself out if I tried to be everything for Brian. One of my weaknesses has been an overarching belief that I can do it all! A few weeks into this new phase of our life, I had one of those epiphanies that made me realize I needed to get some outside help.

One morning, Brian was sleeping late and I wanted to go to a nearby gym to work out, so I decided to leave him a note. We've all seen caricatures of someone who speaks only English, but speaks very slowly and loudly to a foreign-language-speaking person in the vain hope that somehow that will enable him to understand. It never works, and the same concept didn't work for me now. In my effort to help Brian, I wrote my message in big block letters—so large that the note required several pieces of paper, which I carefully taped to the front door. I ran to get my keys, but when I got back to the door, I came to a sudden stop. The realization hit me hard. No matter how large the letters, Brian couldn't read them. I burst into tears, went back into the kitchen, made myself a cup of tea (it's the Irish version of chicken soup—we think it cures everything!), and told myself that this would get better. I had to believe that Brian would improve. And while he did progress because of his determined efforts, it did take a while. I came to realize that I could not do it all. I needed to find someone to help with his speech therapy exercises and facilitate all of his continuing projects by reading things to him. I came up with the idea of hiring a student at a college located near our home. Hiring college and high school students turned out to have many positives, as we found our "helpers" to be fresh young minds who, as an added bonus, were computer literate. My only complaint has been how quickly the time flies: it seems that each student gets to the point of graduating and moving on with his own life far more quickly than we are ready for.

This type of valuable assistance is worth looking into. It's as beneficial to the wife/husband/advocate as it is to the patient—I know that I'd have been a victim of big-time burnout without this help. So look into the resources available in your community; they could be as close to you as the high school student across the street.

Advocate Tip
#45

Access Community Services

It's crucial that you get as much help as you can for your patient and yourself. Every community has services that will assist you and your patient with everything from helping with transportation to reading for the blind. Every hospital or rehabilitation facility has a social worker who can get you started. They can also help you answer questions you may have about Social Security benefits for patients deemed disabled for the long term and short term. See page 215 for resources specifically related to aphasia.

Independence was an important goal for Brian when it came to aphasia, and that's where I could help. Watching someone robbed of much of his dignity while he's in the doctor's office or a hospital is something that bothers me a great deal. But it was far easier to make sure that Brian was given a nightshirt that would cover his 6-foot-3 frame than it has been to help him maintain his pride and his dignity throughout this long-term battle against aphasia. This was a man who was able to keep a jury listening to his every word. Now, he was struggling to find each and every word he said, as well as each and every word he read. For years, someone had to read everything to him. It was incredibly time-consuming, as we often had to read and reread to him so that he could be certain that he clearly understood the material. I agreed that it was essential to keep him informed on what was going on around him.

Brian can now read almost anything if given the time. It's just that in this rushed and hectic world, sometimes you aren't given any time. It's interesting. If you see someone with a cane or in a wheelchair, you know they have trouble walking, and so you make exceptions for them. If their arm is held at a funny angle, you know that they have probably suffered a stroke. We are all willing to make exceptions for, and even help, those whose abilities have been diminished. Or rather, those whose abilities we can *see* have been diminished. That's the problem. We all expect everyone to be able to read, and I think there is an inherent belief in many of us that those who can't read are stupid, or somehow not worthy of our help. There's an old saying my grandmother taught me: "There, but for the grace of God, go I." It behooves all of us to remember that the person standing in front of you at the post office who misspeaks or can't read something may well have been a neurosurgeon just a few months ago.

Brian has improved so much that we no longer have to use many of the tricks we developed when the going was rough, but we have already incorporated many of them into our daily lives, and we do them without thinking.

I wake up much earlier than Brian, and by the time he's up, I've read the newspaper and have tagged items that I read to him. At this point, he can struggle through the newspaper, put much of an article into context, and come up with its meaning, but if I'm around, it's much quicker if I just read things to him. When we check into a hotel, we go up to the counter together and I'll turn to Brian and say, "Do you want me to check in while you go see if they are still serving lunch?" (or whatever excuse I come up with at that moment). At a doctor's office, or whenever he's given a form to fill out, I'll just take it and say, "He's just so spoiled. He hates to do paperwork." Early on in this problem phase, Brian would look at a menu and practice giving his order, but when the waiter came up to the table, he'd freeze and be unable to say anything. When I saw his look of panic, I would say, "Are you still planning on having the scallops?" When it comes to paying or tipping waiters, or bellmen or taxi drivers, I always figure out what they're owed and slip that amount of money to Brian. It would be just as easy for me to pay it myself, but it saves his dignity and pride if he appears to do it all himself.

When we're watching any sports events and they put information up on the screen or JumboTron, I read it aloud.

I'm sure that the people around us must think that I'm some little ditz with my comments like, "Oh, I didn't know that the Patriots had won thirteen games." I didn't realize that this has become an ingrained habit until I was visiting my sister, Carol, in Atlanta a few months ago. We were watching television and without thinking, I was reading out loud anything I saw written in the scroll at the bottom of the screen. Until she stopped me, I was unaware that I was even doing it. These are the little things I do, and it seems a small price to pay for giving Brian the gift of pride. He deserves it, and so much more.

Advocate Tip
#46

Help Maintain Your Patient's Dignity

When people become patients, their health is not the only thing they lose; they can easily lose their dignity, too. As an advocate, you can and should help ensure that your patient's independence and pride are preserved as much as possible. From reading aloud in a casual way for someone who can't, to offering a subtle "hand-up" to a person whose mobility is compromised, think of all the little things you can do to help your loved one maintain dignity—and do them.

Brian

The work of adjusting to the aftereffects of my cancer is grueling. If you've been the victim of a stroke or had to recover from any serious physical trauma, you've faced your own challenges and you know what I mean. I can see progress, but of course there have been setbacks. There were times when I embarrassed myself as a result of my unbridled optimism. In early December of 2000, Gerri and I were at a dinner with the Hastings law school board of directors when I stood up to tell one of my Irish jokes, a joke I had told a hundred times before. Well, the telling of a joke requires not only timing, but a memory of the joke's punchline. I had neither that night. Honestly, beyond the very first line of the joke, I could not come up with another word. It was humiliating. I have always feared embarrassing myself, and that night I realized that I had pushed myself too far, too fast. Luckily, Gerri was sitting by my side and since she had heard that same joke many times before, she was able to feed me line after line of the joke until we had completed our version of Edgar Bergen and Charlie McCarthy. When I retold this event to my speech therapist the following week, she remarked that one of the things allowing me to make progress was that instead of letting an experience like this send me into the depths of despair, I just got very angry at myself and vowed to work harder. Suffer embarrassment? Yes. Give up? Never!

Gerri

While your patient deserves all the kudos he or she gets, as an advocate, you may not receive many yourself along the way. Yes, you will have received the ultimate gift of making a difference in the life of a loved one. Still, in many ways you will be the unseen member of the team. You won't be the one getting the high fives; hopefully, you'll be giving them. There won't be celebrations held in your honor; hopefully, you'll be putting parties together. People won't be coming up to you and telling you how wonderful you are, or even how great you look. Few people other than another advocate will really understand the pressure you've been under. Or how you've put your life on hold. Or how exhausted you are. Your struggle is not something you will—or should—share beyond your closest friends or family, because you know that no matter how you phrase it, it sounds like whining or complaining. One of the best things you can do for yourself in this regard is to find someone else who has been an advocate.

Reach Out to Other Advocates

Advocate Tip
#**47**

Find someone who has "been there, done that," and you'll find that you have an empathetic shoulder to lean on when you need it most. Through your hospital social worker or the organization that relates to the specific illness you are dealing with, you can find numerous support groups. I have friends who've joined these groups and found them truly helpful.

If you're not one to join a group, make sure that you find someone who can understand what you are going through, someone you can talk to when you're feeling overwhelmed, someone who has been an advocate. You won't have to search hard. You will probably find that someone who's been through what you're going through will reach out to you. It might be a good friend. It might even be someone you'd never have thought of as a friend. But this is a time when you will find that a helping hand will reach out to you and buoy you up. Accept that help and be ready to keep the circle going, by reaching out to the next advocate you meet.

Brian

You may find it hard to believe that a big lug like me has a strong sense of the romantic, but I do. Now that my courtroom battles are over, the truth can be told. One of my favorite characters of all time is Cyrano de Bergerac. In my desire to regain independence, I've often thought about the wonderful scene when Cyrano stood looking out a window, giving his famous white plume soliloquy: "I stand not high, it may be, but alone." It's hard for me to convey my supreme need for independence, "to sing, to laugh, to dream, to walk in my own way" and "never to make a line I have not heard in my own heart." But if you're undergoing serious illness, I know you'll understand.

I may have thought of myself as Cyrano in the past, but the reality is that during this time I was very dependent on Gerri. With the arrival of cancer I desperately needed an advocate. And with the arrival of aphasia, my advocate needed enormous patience. With my aphasia, Gerri's responsibilities became greatly magnified. To Gerri, I borrow from Cyrano in saying, "I thank you! And again, I thank you!"

Chapter Ten

RECOGNIZE THE GIFTS YOU'VE BEEN GIVEN

*Dance as if no one were watching, sing as if no one were listening,
and live every day as if it were your last.*
—AN IRISH BLESSING

Gerri

Cancer patients are traditionally given the five-year cancer-free marker as something to aim for. That five-year mark is seen by many as the bellwether for success in fighting their cancer, and it usually is. But Brian at five years was so far beyond the norm for metastatic melanoma with two brain metastases that no one was able to tell me whether this really was an all-clear or not. As one doctor told me, "I don't know how he got this far, so I can't tell you how far he can go."

We decided to celebrate it anyhow.

I put together an invitation that read, "Five years later. We have been blessed with so many gifts during the past five years. Each and every day. Five beautiful grandchildren. The best physicians and medical care available. A continuing clean bill of health. And, not least of all . . . laughter and the love of friends."

It was a great party, and more important, a wonderful celebration of life.

Brian

Actually, it was an Irish wake. You may have figured out by now that the Irish often have a weird sense of humor, and that holds true for a longtime friend of mine, Judge Gerry Lewis. About a year or so into my fight with cancer, when it appeared that I was not in imminent danger of losing the battle, a bunch of my friends were gathered at our local watering hole. They were all marveling at the fact that I was still there, standing right beside them. With his always puckish humor, Judge Lewis told me that when they had first heard my diagnosis, he and The Lads began planning an outstanding Irish wake for me. The idea was to have a great party, full of laughter, singing, drinking, and many stories told about me. But I had ruined their plans. As Gerry put it, "Monaghan, we're happy that you're here. But there is a downside. We had been planning a great party in your honor. You sure spoiled that!"

Gerri and I were happy to call the judge at the five-year mark and tell him that the wake would go on as originally planned with one great exception—I was going to be in attendance! It doesn't get much better for me than to bask in the affection and love of good family and friends. Once again, I reflected on how lucky I have been—lucky enough to be on the receiving end of so much love, lucky enough to have been able to attend my own funeral and wake.

Our house is small but built around several patios, and the walls are mostly glass, so when close friends are jammed in it makes for good times. Gerri had decorated the place with photographs of me: one in my "navy whites," another with my two brothers in our football uniforms when we played together in high school, some of me with Kathi and Patrick when they were young. There were photos of Gerri's and my wedding, which had taken place in this very house. There were lots of photos from trips we'd taken.

Gerri isn't one to let me take myself too seriously, so she'd also placed a life-size picture of me dressed up as Miss Piggy for all to see when they first walked in. This had been my Halloween costume back in 1997—replete with pig nose, big eyelashes, a blond wig with a big black bow on top, and a pink tutu (it said one size fits all but if that elastic snapped, I could have done someone major damage). Anyhow, this was the main poster people saw when they got to the front door, so most of them were laughing when they walked in. A lot of the guests had been at our wedding eight years earlier. Many, too, found themselves in the photos she'd scattered all around the house, so that brought comments like, "Do you remember that trip? Wasn't that the time we . . ." I think it's safe to say a good time was had by all.

This was such a special night, one which, once again, made me appreciate the "gift of cancer."

Celebrate the Milestones

Advocate Tip
48

Brian and I both believe that it makes far more sense to spend money on a party than a funeral. Whether it's ending a round of chemotherapy or radiation, or reaching any other medical milestone, recognizing the value of the achievement gives your patient a huge psychological boost. Even if the accomplishment seems insignificant, it's likely that it involved painful procedures, tough times, and enormous effort. It's not just about overcoming the odds: think of the fear and discouragement that nibbles around the edges of every patient's thoughts. When your loved one has rounded some corner in the battle, a reward is in order. I recommend celebrating. Although my husband is always ready for a lively party, your patient may not be. No matter. It doesn't have to be a grand affair. A potluck dinner with a few close friends can be all the recognition called for. But do recognize each milestone. Every one is important.

Brian

I often reflect on the words Gerri said to me on that first day when we left Dan Einhorn's office: "Bear, however long we have, whatever time we have, we are going to deal with this with two things . . . laughter and love. I'm willing to bet that in whatever time we have left, people we know will die in car accidents or keel over from heart attacks. We are going to have the ability to cherish and really appreciate each and every day. We are going to love and laugh and fight this . . . and you are going to win."

It's been more than ten years since I got my diagnosis, and these years are an amazing gift. I wouldn't be here without the love and support of Gerri and so many, many others. Being around to "feel the love" is a gift that keeps on giving. It happens every time I run into a former client who grabs my hand and says, "Thanks again for all you did for me." It happens when an attorney pulls me aside and says, "I watched you in trial dozens of times and I learned so much from you." It happens each time a person comes up to me and says, "You don't know me, but I know who you are. Years ago, one of your clients was my best friend and you really helped her. I've prayed for you often. I still do and I'm so happy that I've finally been able to meet you and can tell you this." Wow! Am I lucky or what?

I've been given far more time than anyone ever believed possible. Gerri was right: friends did die while we continued to fight our own battle. Brave and wonderful fellow patients I met along the way lost their struggles with cancer, and several other friends have died of it as well. Other friends are now fighting the disease themselves.

But there have been unforeseen delights, too. I have grown closer to Gerri's children. I have come to rely on them at times, and I have come to understand and be comforted by the fact that without a doubt, Todd and Mark would always take great care of their mother. Our seven amazing grandchildren, who might have come to know me only through photos and stories, have been a special bonus I appreciate more with each passing day. New friends entered into our lives. Some of our hopes fizzled, but others surged. We've traveled, particularly to places that Gerri had not seen and that we could share together.

Throughout it all, Gerri and I began to understand that while a life-changing or terminal illness may be brutal, it is in fact a gift, whether the time left to us is short or long. Twenty years ago, when one friend had died and another had been horribly burned in an airplane accident, I heard this very same message and thought I understood it. But until cancer struck, I hadn't really comprehended the message at all. I'm not naïve enough to think that my words will have any kind of an impact on someone who is not facing a life-threatening situation, because I'm not sure that any of us can really understand this lesson until we are smacked in the face, dealing with our own mortality. But like those who came before me and offered the same words of advice, while I may not be able to convince you, I can tell you what I've learned.

I have come to understand and appreciate that I was given the time to take care of my family as best I could. The person who dies in a car crash, or suffers a fatal heart attack or some other sudden event, often leaves everything in the hands of other people (usually their family). The survivors are not only mentally crushed by this sudden tragedy, but in the midst of it, are forced to deal with the complexities of arranging a funeral and organizing family matters as well as any business dealings the departed may have. With the gift of extra time, that shouldn't happen to you.

Extra time gives you the opportunity to close doors that must be closed, and open other doors. This is the time when you can allow yourself the luxury of saying, "Life's too short to spend time with people I don't like, or doing things I don't like." As you stand facing the reality that you are closer to death than you had ever really understood before, issues become clearer. Facing death can often give us crystal clear vision. If you have been given the gift of attending your own funeral, you will understand that this is now your turn to reach out to others and let them hear words of love or appreciation from you. It becomes far easier to say, "Thanks, my friend," or, "I love you." It's also a time for healing old wounds. "I'm truly, truly sorry"—words you once thought you would choke over—come rolling off your tongue. The argument that might have burdened a relationship suddenly seems inconsequential, and this gift of time you have been given allows you to correct it.

Only when I was in immediate danger of losing it did I learn to appreciate the wonder of life. I would be lying if I told you

167

that in the last ten years, I have focused on and truly enjoyed every minute of every day. It's really discouraging for me to realize that too often there have been times when I began to lose that appreciation. I've found myself watching inane television shows or doing other worthless activities. I remember a story in one of Ernest Hemingway's books that told of a WWI soldier in a foxhole with bombs exploding all around him. He curled up in a ball and prayed passionately to God. He vowed that he would never sin again if God would only allow him to survive. Somehow, he made it through that night, but when the bombing ended at sunrise he went to town, got drunk, and found himself a prostitute. It's all too easy for this gift to slip away. Whenever I find that happening to me, I ask myself, "What the hell am I doing?" That helps remind me of the gift I have been given. As a longtime friend, Dr. Arch Woodard, has often reminded me: "Suck the marrow out of each day."

Gerri

Brian is obviously far more noble than I. When he first began talking about the "gift of cancer," I asked him if it would be possible to regift it.

But I do recognize the gifts we've been given. How could I not? How could I not recognize the gifts I've been given? First is the gift of being the advocate for a man who always looks at the glass as half full, a man for whom optimism is second nature. Fighting the battle against any disease can be debilitating for the advocate as well as the patient, and I count my lucky stars that I've shared this struggle with someone who has appreciated each and every thing I have done to help him. Believe me, that's a huge mark in the plus column.

I've been blessed with ten years of sharing Christmas together—when I started out hoping and praying for just one more. The gifts I've been given are many. The gift of toasting each other every night with the words, "Aren't we lucky?" Sharing life with our grandchildren has been the best of all gifts. The gift of watching Brian taking Trevor's hand as they walk into the baseball park to see the Padres play, and then to watch Brian break into a grin when he hears Trevor recite all the players' names by heart. The gift of watching Brian swell with pride as Kyra reads her books to him, or snuggles against his shoulder. The gift of hearing him growl at Reagan, "What's your name, kid?" and hearing him roar with laughter when this five-year-old looks up at him from a two-foot disadvantage and growls back, "You want a piece of me?" The gift of watching giant sized "Poppa" sit next to Cassidy on teeny little chairs, drinking her pretend tea from tiny pink cups. The gift of watching him pace up and down the soccer or baseball or football field, cheering Riley on, or teaching him to play gin rummy. The gift of watching Brian's face light up with joy as Dylan gets a hit and runs as fast as he can to first base. And knowing that there will be gifts to share with Jake as well.

It's a gift to know that as an advocate, I really did play a big part in helping to get him here. And there are gifts that will come your way in the battle you're facing, though sometimes, they may be difficult to find. And yes, there are days (many days) when you, too, will want to regift!

One of my favorite sayings has always been "Enjoy life. This is not a dress rehearsal." It's something I had to remind myself of many times during the past ten years. I found that one of the most difficult things for an advocate to do is to let go. Have you ever seen the overprotective mother, hovering around the child who's experienced some health problem? Not just hovering, but constantly telling him that he's incapable of doing or trying new things? You can certainly understand where the mother is coming from, but it's also easy to see how destructive her behavior can be in the long run.

This often happens with an advocate. You work so hard to achieve the success that has kept your patient alive a little bit longer, that there's often a tendency to want to protect them from anything that might go wrong. But he or she is not living each day to the fullest if you keep your patient wrapped up in some kind of cocoon, hoping to prevent anything from going wrong. It's not living if your patient isn't allowed to enjoy life.

Remember, This Is Not a Dress Rehearsal

Yes, you need to make sure he takes his medicines or has his checkups, and you take away as much stress from his life as you can, but there's only so much you can do. You will never be able to control everything. So if your patient has always wanted to take a special trip, after making sure it's okay with his doctor, go for it. Even if it means cutting life short by a day or a week or a month or a year, isn't it better to have enjoyed that life? Remind yourself that this is not a dress rehearsal. Let your loved one live to the fullest extent possible, rather than languishing in the wings, simply waiting for the curtain to fall.

Brian

When Lou Gehrig was honored on the field of Yankee Stadium as the greatest first baseman who ever played, his career had just come to an end. He had been diagnosed with Amyotrophic Lateral Sclerosis (ALS), an incurable, progressive neurodegenerative disease that affects the ability of the brain to initiate and control muscle movement. When the speeches were finished and the gifts presented, the time came for him to respond. A very shy man, Lou was finally coaxed by the crowd to step up and speak. He said simply, "For the past two weeks you've been reading about the bad break I got. Yet, today, I consider myself the luckiest man on the face of this earth. I have been in ballparks for seventeen years and have never received anything but kindness and encouragement from you fans. . . . Sure, I'm lucky. When you have a wife who has been a tower of strength and shown more courage than you dreamed existed— that's the finest I know. So I close in saying that I may have had a tough break, but I have an awful lot to live for."

And when the great trial lawyer Louis "Louie" Nizer was asked how he had been "so lucky in the courtroom" throughout his career, Nizer responded that "most of his luck came late at night in a law library."

In various ways, many people have asked me how it is that I am still alive. I occasionally have flippantly said, "Maybe it was just luck." But that was clearly not the case. The true answer is, I have been given a gift that is one part Gehrig's "luck," one part Nizer's "luck," and two parts Gerri Monaghan.

How have I survived? Was it merely a series of coincidences that helped me win this fight? How did it all happen to come together? I know that I didn't do this on my own. I was helped in so many ways, by so many people. To each and every one of you, thank you for your help, thank you for your prayers, your laughter, and your love. This battle against cancer has made it difficult for me to think that there is not a God. How could there not be?

A friend of mine was right: "The Holy Bench has given me a continuance." And my thanks for that continuance has to take the form of paying it forward, reaching out to the next person, extending my hand in friendship to them. Gerri and I do that; we are always willing to help in any way we can, hence this attempt to help others through this book. I hope we've been able to reach you with our message. Fight whatever disease or medical problem you have with all you've got, and make sure you've got a strong advocate by your side. Go on the offense. Push the envelope. Revel in the laughter and love of friends. And recognize that facing your own mortality can give you the gift of appreciating life as many can't.

Gerri

No one knows why Brian has survived his stage IV melanoma. I don't have the answer, and I've been there every step of the way. Surely, some of it has been pure blind luck. Don't forget— this is the guy who could beat me at cards while still in the ICU after brain surgery! But I don't believe you can trace the answer to coincidence. I guess I don't really believe in coincidences. I think so much of this can be better explained by phrases like "what goes around, comes around" or "karma" or "six degrees of separation" or "paying it forward." However you choose to explain it, his story does seem to defy conventional medical beliefs and perhaps that does qualify his recovery as "miraculous."

From a practical standpoint, a great deal of that miracle can be traced back to the fact that Brian is a good man who, during his lifetime, has often reached out to help others. And when he got sick and needed help, his good deeds came back to him. Full circle. The people whose lives he had touched in the past were people who, in turn, reached out to him.

We have been given so many gifts in the past ten years. While writing this book has been our major attempt to pay those gifts forward, something else we can do in that regard is to give *you* the gift of hope, the gift of learning to not accept no as an answer, the gift of not giving up too soon, the gift of understanding that statistics and numbers often lie, the gift of knowing that there's always the exception to the rule. You deserve the chance to hope that you are that exception!

Hope does exist, but not in a vacuum. Hope requires help. Your help. Hope lies in the research labs where scientists are seeking cures for various diseases. But you have to help find those medical advances. Hope lies in the newest medical treatments and cutting-edge technology. But you have to be the one to seek out those treatments. Hope cannot exist without your help.

Always Think in Terms of "We"

Not until I was proofreading our manuscript did I notice something important, something I had never thought of before. From the very beginning, the word "we" has been at the forefront. When "we" had the Gamma Knife. When "we" went to Dallas for the vaccine. When "we" were dealing with the brain seizures. As an advocate, I thought of myself as part of a team. I never saw this as Brian's battle, with me serving as an attentive cheerleader. We were fighting this together. It was our battle. It was our war. I know that in many ways, we won it together. There's no denying that Brian was the one who felt the pain, was on the operating table, and lived through this every minute of every day. But as far as it was humanly possible, his fight was my fight. In looking back at the last ten years, I think that concept is a truly worthy one. If, as the advocate, you can really feel that this is your war, you will realize that no one has a more vested interest in winning than you do.

Well, we did it. Brian and I are still together, even after the arduous task of writing a book *together!* It wasn't easy, but I would not be telling you the truth if I said that the last ten years have been easy. They haven't.

Yes, it has been difficult, but it's a difficulty I can handle. In June of 1998, I was praying that Brian would be around just six more months. Since then, I've had the sublime joy of watching seven beautiful grandchildren jump into the arms of their beloved "Poppa Bri." We've shared great laughs with great friends, and shared tears as we've lost other friends to our No. 1 foe, cancer. Throughout it all, I have maintained my role as advocate. I know I have made a big contribution in the life of the man I love, and boy, has he been worth saving. His spirit is larger than life and whatever tough times there have been, they are more than made up for by the fact that he's still here by my side. Has it been tough? You bet. Would I go through it again? As this girl from the Bronx would say, in a New York minute.

Ten years ago, I told Brian that we would approach this journey with laughter and love and that we would push the envelope to get him the medical help he needed. We've done that. What's more, not a day goes by that we don't tell each other how fortunate, how blessed, how very lucky we are. We hope that your journey will be as successful, and that you will be able to come to appreciate that you can find the positive in even serious illness, if you look hard enough. And don't forget . . . pay it forward!

Brian

If I could give everyone reading this a gift, it would be the gift of living life to the very fullest, embracing the world and everything in it as you fight with all you've got to hang on tight.

Flashback to my "funeral" at our house five years ago. The party is in full swing. Friends and family are laughing, sharing Monaghan stories, and I've never been happier to be ribbed by them all. Suddenly, I hear the deep, warm voice of Louis

Armstrong singing *our song*, "What a Wonderful World," the song we had chosen for the first dance at our wedding. It's a moment I want to share with Gerri but our home is packed with family and friends and it takes me a while to find her. As I look for her, I find myself humming along, the lyrics once again resonating with me. In the past five years, I have seen babies cry and I've watched them grow—my grandchildren. I've seen seasons come and go. I've lived a wonderful life over the past five years. Just as I reach Gerri, the song is about to end, but as I wrap her in my arms there's time for me to sing along with Louis the last two iconic words . . .

"Oh, yeah!"

EPILOGUE

Whatsoever thy hand findeth to do, do it with thy might;
For there is no work, nor device, nor knowledge,
nor wisdom in the grave where thou goest.

—ECCLESIASTES 9:10

Brian

In late May 2005, Gerri and I took a vacation to Normandy, France. We thought of this trip as a reward to ourselves, and not just for my having lived six years longer than anyone thought possible. At this point we had completed much of the work on the project we had embraced as our mission—this book—and the trip was a way of congratulating ourselves. We hoped our attempt to pay it forward would help others faced with a life-threatening disease.

Our experience in Normandy made us understand that we still had a long way to go.

The morning after our arrival, Gerri and I walked along Omaha Beach. Of the various beaches utilized in the D-Day invasion of World War II, Omaha was particularly significant. Thousands of young men had gone ashore at this very spot, and too many had lost their lives to the bullets raining down on them from the machine gun emplacements above. But now, as we walked along, it was eerily silent. We heard no gunfire, no cries of pain, no calls for medics. It was peaceful, completely quiet except for the sound of the lapping of waves from the North Atlantic. On this early morning, there were only a few other people on the beach, and most of them were white-haired, bent over their canes, apparently reliving their experiences from the war.

Gerri and I both love history and we knew that the D-Day invasion was one of the seminal events of our lifetime, so we had done a lot of research, reading as many books and watching as many films on WWII as we could. We thought we were prepared for Normandy, and in the historical sense we were. But on an emotional level, what we experienced was something for which we were not prepared at all.

As we stood there, I could hear in my mind the sounds from the scenes in the movies we had watched. The sounds of young men, dying brutally. I knew that this beach represented the end of life for thousands of them. They had been kids from small towns and big cities. Farm boys from Chappell, Nebraska, and truck drivers from Chicago. Young lawyers from Boston, and ranch hands from Butte, Montana. I've learned that sixty-plus years later, most of the D-Day survivors can still recall the names of the men who died alongside them. For me, walking down Omaha Beach brought a powerful realization that too many young men's hopes and dreams ended in a matter of seconds as they touched the sands of a distant country. The brutality of it all was something I found incomprehensible.

Later in the day, we visited the American Cemetery—row upon row of starkly white crosses, marking 9,387 graves. A magnificent bronze statue, "Spirit of American Youth," towers above it all. Walking in this cemetery was like nothing I have ever experienced. I felt as if I were in an enormous outdoor cathedral, and the dignity and solemnity of the place moved me deeply. With tears in her eyes, Gerri whispered that she wished each of the mothers of those buried here had been able to come so she could understand that her boy was now in hallowed ground. We weren't the only ones affected. Walking between the rows of the cemetery was a large group of French schoolchildren. There was no pushing or shoving, no joking. They walked along in silence. I was struck by this as I could not recall ever having seen a group of children so completely silent. Even those young children understood that they were in a sacred place.

As neither Gerri nor I had any relatives buried in Normandy, she suggested that we merely select the name of a Monaghan and find his grave. Peter Monaghan's grave was near the end of a row in section D. From where we stood, we could hear the sounds of the North Atlantic. A few rows away was the grave of a brigadier general, Theodore Roosevelt, Jr., the son of our twenty-sixth president. Officers, enlisted men, Jewish, Catholic, Protestant, boys from all over the U.S. All killed. Each of those kids must have had his own story, how he lived, how he died, what dreams he might have had. All gone.

As Gerri and I stood by these graves, once again all was silence. A flood of thoughts raged through me. So many deaths. All so young. I thought about promises not kept, and lost possibilities. What could these young men have achieved if they had lived? Did the cure for cancer lie buried here? Or the final understanding of Alzheimer's or Parkinson's? Or a brilliant technological discovery of some kind? We'll never know. Anger and frustration welled up within me. Then came the tears. I thought about the fact that I was a sixty-six-year-old man who for some unknown reason was alive when I was supposed to have been dead years before. I couldn't make any sense of it.

When we got home, I sank into a rare depression. I kept asking myself, "Why me? Why am I still alive when so many young kids lost their lives before they even started to live?" I've never been able to come up with a good answer. The simple, "Why *not* me?" was the only thing that made any sense.

I've never been introspective. I've always had the ability, or maybe the need, to turn gloomy thoughts into something positive. The anger, despair, and frustration brought on by my trip to Normandy gave way to a burning need to just *do something*. I thought about the survivors of the war and the responsibilities our country had toward them. I decided that as a cancer survivor, it was my responsibility to do more. Writing this book wasn't enough. In order to pay it forward, I needed to become more involved in the war on cancer. As a survivor, I could and should do no less.

I'm no medical expert, but I do know that because there are more than 200 different types of cancer, finding a "cure for cancer" will be difficult. I've heard doctors and scientists say that they don't expect to find a cure, but rather a way to somehow contain it. They want it to be as treatable as a chronic illness. But damn it, that's not good enough. Walking on the moon was difficult, too! Back in 1962, I'd heard President John F. Kennedy's speech when he issued a challenge to our country:

"We choose to go to the moon. We choose to go to the moon in this decade and do other things, not because they are easy, but because they are hard, because that goal will serve to organize and measure the best of our energies and skills, because that challenge is one that we are willing to accept, one we are unwilling to postpone, and one which we intend to win. . . ."

Although Kennedy didn't live to see men walk on the moon, the work on meeting that challenge continued to move forward and was accomplished seven years later, in 1969. Those of us who are cancer patients and survivors are not insisting that a cure for this disease be accomplished in time for us to benefit personally. But damn it, we'd like to know that there will be a cure for our children and our grandchildren.

It was way back in January 1971, during a State of the Union address, that President Richard Nixon requested an additional $100 million for cancer research:

"The time has come in America when the same kind of concentrated effort that split the atom and took man to the moon should be turned to conquering dread disease. Let us make a total national commitment to achieve this goal."

In December 1971, Nixon signed the National Cancer Act. As a nation, we had officially declared war on cancer.

Yet, thirty-seven years later, that war isn't close to being won. Ask any of the half million people who were diagnosed with cancer last year if they feel like they're a winner. Ask the millions of families who've buried loved ones who lost their battle against cancer if they believe this is a war that's been won. They know it hasn't been won. So the question becomes, why not?

Why hasn't this war been won? Where's the commitment? Where's the anger?

Yes, progress has been made on many fronts. Since the war on cancer was declared there have been amazing advances in detection, prevention, and treatment. In the past, receiving a diagnosis of cancer was seen as a virtual death sentence, but now more than half of all cancer patients are still alive at the five-year mark. In 1990, with the help of funding from the National Institutes of Health (NIH) and the Department of Energy, a gigantic step forward was made: the Human Genome Project began. Scientists believe that attacking the genetic roots of diseases such as Alzheimer's, Parkinson's, diabetes, and cancer will lead to new methods of diagnosis, prevention, and treatment. The project's completion in 2003 marked a very hopeful step, but it will take years before scientists are able to turn this newly acquired knowledge into something concrete to help the thousands of people afflicted with these diseases. It will take more than time—it will take money. Lots of it. As we complete this book at the end of 2008, our country faces a huge economic crisis. This is bound to cause even more of a struggle to obtain federal funding. But we cannot abandon these projects. We must move ahead.

The need for federal funding is vital. The NIH is the primary agency for conducting and supporting medical research; its track record in improving the health of our nation's citizens is impressive. As citizens, we should expect—and insist—that the NIH continue at the frontlines of medical research, which will benefit all of us, not just cancer patients. The only way that progress can continue is with enough funding on the federal level.

Although federal funding for the NIH doubled between 1997 and 2003, since then the funding levels have increased only marginally, with many scientists arguing that, due to inflation, the funding has actually decreased in terms of real dollars. In May 2008, a group of high-powered university presidents and professors testified before a Senate panel. They compiled a report indicating that in real dollars, the purchasing power of the NIH had decreased 13 percent since 2003. They argued for a significant increase in funding for the NIH. In addition, they expressed their concern that the lack of funding for research grants from the NIH will lead to a "brain drain" that could have a long-lasting impact on the health of our citizenry. If nine out of ten young research scientists who apply for grants are turned down due to lack of sufficient funding, these scientists are likely either to leave academic research entirely or to take their research to countries more supportive of their efforts.

Let me state it again. The money going into federally funded research has *decreased* 13 percent since 2003. Remember, "federally funded" means that's *our* money. More than half a million of our citizens died last year from cancer alone. And the funding has gone down. Where is the outrage? I'm outraged and you should be as well.

As a beneficiary of cutting-edge medical research and technology myself, maybe I should just be quiet and thank my lucky stars. But I can't do that. Not if I want our children and grandchildren to benefit from even newer medical advances.

When I returned from Normandy, I stumbled along, trying to come up with a vehicle to accomplish this goal. For years, Gerri and I have been supporters of fund-raisers devoted to cancer research and other diseases, and we applaud everyone who gets involved at their local community level in doing this. We also applaud the good work done by volunteers in local organizations, such as the American Cancer Society or the American Heart Association. These volunteers do everything they can to extend a helping hand to those who are afflicted with the same disease from which the volunteers have recovered. And we strongly admire those who volunteer to work with Alzheimer's patients or those who work at their local Veterans Administration to help the wounded soldiers returning from war. Each of these volunteers is doing work that is vitally needed.

But personally, I wanted to go in a different direction.

As usual, Gerri listened to my ranting and raving, and between us we came up with the idea for something we called a Citizens Cancer Lobby. Statistics have told us that ten million people are affected by cancer, and that's just those who are diagnosed. For each cancer patient, there's a mother or husband or grandchild or caregiver or advocate, so that ten million expands exponentially. A lobby of all of these people could be extremely powerful.

While I have great passion for this subject, I soon learned that I wasn't the only one to come up with this idea. The American Cancer Society (ACS) was way ahead of me. Everyone has heard of the ACS. Its war against cancer is well known, and the society has proven an invaluable resource for anyone fighting this disease (see page 211 for more on their work).

ACS has helped to achieve some of the enormous success in the fight against cancer, but beginning in 2001, their leadership decided to go in a new direction. They decided they needed more political muscle. They created a new entity, a political action organization known as ACS CAN (American Cancer Society Cancer Action Network), with the mandate to engage in policy analysis, direct lobbying of politicians, grassroots action, media outreach, and even litigation to achieve their advocacy goals. These activities culminated in the September 20, 2006, event "Celebration on the Hill," in which more than 10,000 individuals gathered in Washington, D.C., rallied on Capitol Hill, and lobbied legislators to get involved in the fight against cancer. In the past year, I have become an "ambassador" for ACS CAN and recently went to meet with and lobby our local senate and assembly representatives in Sacramento, to ask for more funding for cancer research and patient access to health care. It's about time that we demanded that cancer victims have a say in how our tax dollars are spent.

ACS CAN also decided to take a stand on holding politicians accountable. During the recent election, they asked major party candidates in federal and state races around the country to state with specificity where they stood on high-priority cancer issues. Candidates were asked what they would do to support more funding for cancer research as well as what they would do to work toward meaningful health care reforms. ACS CAN has hundreds of thousands of volunteers in congressional districts across the nation who are willing to hold our elected officials accountable and determine if their votes on these issues are consistent with their answers prior to their election.

One person *can* make a difference in this war. In recent years, a hero of mine, Lance Armstrong, has become a cancer activist, arguing for the need for increased federal funding. In 2005 he met with President George Bush, who asked Lance what he needed in his fight against cancer. Armstrong replied, "A billion dollars." He followed up with a letter to the president, saying, "It's time for a bold initiative to combat this disease, which kills 560,000 Americans every year." While Armstrong received words of praise and encouragement, no initiative or further funding was forthcoming.

Armstrong then changed course. He began to get involved in politics. Not partisan politics of Democrat versus Republican. The politics of cancer. Armstrong went to Iowa, a pivotal political state, and began discussing the issue of raising the fight against cancer as a national priority for voters. He announced his intention to start a movement to bring cancer to the forefront of voters' minds. He has held forums and political debates during which candidates for public office are asked their views on funding cancer research. He continues to stay neutral and apolitical, but Armstrong's support of any candidate will now be made on the basis of that individual's stand on the war against cancer. In effect, Lance Armstrong has become a leader of a citizens' lobbying effort.

While few of us have the power or face recognition of Lance Armstrong, we can each be part of that same type of effort. It's time for each of us to become an activist. I'm not talking about taking to the barricades, but I am talking about getting involved. I know that for some, their mission in life might be to play their best golf game ever. Or climb the highest mountain. Or win their next legal battle. But to those of us touched by cancer, or any other life-threatening disease, our mission must be more significant because we have come to understand the precious gift of life. And I believe that as survivors, we have been charged with the task of paying it forward.

Follow Lance Armstrong's lead and make your voice heard. Pick up the phone and call your local congressperson or senator. Find out what his or her position is on federal funding for the NIH or funding for the specific agency on the front lines of whatever disease is of particular interest to you.

Join others in your community who are fighting for the same specific cause you're interested in. Federal funding isn't just about cancer research. We need to find the cause and the cure for Alzheimer's. We need to come up with a treatment for Parkinson's. We need to fund more research into how to overcome devastating brain injuries. Whatever your cause, whatever your passion, it's likely there's a local group in your community involved in the same battle. Call them and find out how you can help.

Can you imagine the effect we would have if we all spoke as one? If just those ten million individuals who have been affected by cancer each picked up the phone and made that call to their congressman, I bet we could tie up the lines for days. By ourselves, our voice is weak, but together, we can be powerful. We can be a potent army in the war against devastating diseases and for the need for health care for all. The gun lobby, the insurance lobby, the pharmaceutical lobby—hundreds of lobbying groups all have their say. But would any of them speak with our numbers, our interest, or our passion?

It's not enough for a politician to say they're "in favor" of cures. It's time for politicians to put *our* money where their mouths are! Because in order to defeat cancer or any other disease, it will be necessary to come up with big bucks. That means taxpayer-funded research. While it's a great idea and worthwhile for each of us to get personally involved, we can run all the 10K races in the world on behalf of our favorite cause and it won't be enough. We can each sponsor ten individuals walking in support of melanoma research but it won't be a drop in the bucket of what we need. We can only win these wars with government funding, and we need to remember that since it really is our money, we should get to have some say in how it's spent.

Which brings me to stem cell research. I've read up on this subject, and listened to lectures by the best researchers in the world. I've had a past president of the California Institute for Regenerative Medicine sit down with paper and pen and draw little circles, patiently trying to explain to me the difference between stem cells made from fertilized eggs and stem cells made from a patient's skin. (I must have slept through Biology 101.)

I may not understand exactly how it works, but I do believe that we are on the cusp of an incredible opportunity: stem cell research may hold the answers for millions of patients with all types of medical problems and diseases. With more than 2,000 research papers on embryonic and adult stem cells published in reputable scientific journals every year, scientists believe that the possibilities for this research are truly endless. Already, adult stem cells are being used in treatments for more than one hundred medical conditions including leukemia and heart disease. So while I don't purport to understand how it works, I do understand that stem cell research offers a magic ingredient missing all too often in our lives. Stem cell research offers hope. Hope for us all.

I'll tip my hat to those who oppose this research. We are all entitled to our political and religious views, and I'm for having scientists and researchers do what they can to be sensitive to the concerns of those in opposition. But I think it's ludicrous to believe that the religious beliefs of a few should hold sway over the lives of millions of Americans. Should such beliefs be allowed to prevent funding the research that might cure Alzheimer's or Parkinson's? Should such beliefs be allowed to control the destiny of a President Reagan or a Michael J. Fox? Or you or me or my grandchildren or yours?

President Obama has taken the first big step, but we must remain vigilant. Find out if your federal representatives are for or against federal funding for stem cell research. If they voted against it, find out the views of the people running against them in the next election, and if their views better represent yours, campaign for them. Vote for them. Make your voice heard.

And one other thing. The efforts of the best scientists in the world, well-funded and producing valuable research that holds the cure for every disease and affliction known to mankind, could all be for naught. It's all just spitting into the wind if patients don't have the ability to get needed treatment. Which brings us to *access* to health care.

Access to health care is the elephant in the room, and I don't think you can begin to discuss any medical issue without acknowledging that too many people in our country are excluded from quality health care. A solution to this problem will require the best work of experts, the dedication of politicians, and nonpartisan cooperation among members of all political parties. I don't have a clue as to how we accomplish the objective of giving everyone access to health care. I just know that somehow, we need to find a way. In its new role as an advocate, ACS CAN has recognized that it's impossible to defeat cancer without a national health care system. So ACS CAN has launched an advertising campaign urging access to health care. In addition, AARP (formerly the American Association of Retired Persons) is now involved in the political arena regarding health care access through its new campaign, "Divided We Fail." This is a large, well-organized group with some strong political clout, and I find their advertisements regarding this to be powerful.

But for most of us, as individuals, it's back to the phone lines. I'm convinced that much of this discussion comes down to political clout. Complaining in private won't do any good at all. This is the time for a call to arms. Each of us needs to get involved. Contact your representatives and ask their positions on access to health care. Listen closely to what is being said in any upcoming election campaign and use this information in making your decision on who should get your vote. Speak up and tell them what you think. Alone, your voice is pretty weak. But remember: you are not alone. Not if each of us decides to speak up, cast our vote, get involved. Realize that you are a part of a citizens' lobby. Your voice can be one of not just thousands, but millions. We can each pay it forward to the next patient who needs a helping hand and by extension, to the next generation. We need only to assume our responsibility and get involved.

This is an exciting time. I believe that thanks to the Human Genome Project and stem cell research, as well as the research at the NIH and other research laboratories across the country, there is a national recognition that now is the time, and we have the ability to achieve our goals.

With Lance Armstrong and his Livestrong Foundation beating the bushes to get support for those candidates for congressional and senatorial offices who agree with their ideas on funding for cancer research, there's hope for the future. With ACS CAN exerting political muscle by meeting with members of Congress and continually demanding increased federal funding for groups like the NIH, there's hope for the future. With groups like AARP advocating on behalf of access to health care, there's hope for the future. And by joining together the voices of those of us afflicted or affected by cancer, or heart disease, or brain damage, or other life-altering disease, there's hope for the future. Maybe not our future, but the future of those we love.

These diseases affect too damned many of us. We need to stand together, to form our own band of brothers and sisters, to unite until the sound of our voices cannot be pushed aside. As an army of survivors, we can be heard.

There is hope. There is much work to be done, but there is hope. For me, personally, I look at the future and say, "Cancer, you son of a bitch, we are coming. And we will win."

THE MONAGHAN MANUAL

We know: most books like ours have appendixes of useful information. But when we looked at what we had to offer, it was so personal, so quirky, that we decided to call it The Monaghan Manual. Our tongues are planted firmly in our cheeks with that title, but still, we're hoping you find this collection useful. It includes websites and phone numbers, Gerri's battle plan and her outline for an Advocate's Notebook, plus books that inspired Brian, some of his favorite (notice, we didn't say tasteful!) Irish jokes, and more. Think of it as a starting-off point as you gather the weapons you'll need to wage and win your own personal battle.

Gerri's Tips at a Glance

We thought you might like to see all fifty of Gerri's advocacy tips at once. Here's a condensed list, cross-referenced to the pages where you'll find the unabridged versions. Feel free to copy this list and tape it inside your own Advocate's Notebook.

Advocate Tip #1 (page 11)

Trust Your Intuition

When there's a little voice inside you insisting that something is wrong, you need to listen to it. Insist on your patient getting checked and checked again.

Advocate Tip #2 (page 14)

Write Down the Medical History

What illnesses and conditions run in your patient's family? Which illnesses has he or she had? What medications is he or she taking and in what dosage? Keep a record and bring it with you to every doctor's appointment.

Advocate Tip #3 (page 18)

Gather Your Courage

Fighting a life-threatening disease is seldom a straight road to success. But with courage, you can get down to the business of making ready for war against a frightening enemy.

Advocate Tip #4 (page 27)

Understand That Advocates Come in Many Forms

Advocates can be adult children, siblings, parents, friends, and even, perhaps, professionals. If you feel that you and your patient need more support, try contacting your local hospitals or the American Cancer Society, Heart Association, or whatever health-related entity you need.

Advocate Tip #5 (page 28)

Don't Let Others' Reactions Get You Down

Talk back when you need to address thoughtless comments, or just brush them off. But don't share them with your patient. Write your "come-backs" down, if only to vent!

Advocate Tip #6 (page 30)

Create a Battle Plan

Your battle plan might vary depending on the situation your loved one is in, but I found that the basics apply across the board, and the very act of forming a plan is helpful. See page 201.

Advocate Tip #7 (page 33)

Keep an Advocate's Notebook

Record names, dates, and places relevant to your patient's health care. Keep phone numbers that you need access to on a constant basis. Keep a chronological record of your patient's appointments and what was done for (or to) him or her. Write down questions you have before appointments.

Advocate Tip #8 (page 36)

Stand Up for Yourself

If your loved one is taking his or her frustration out on you, don't put up with it. Say you are willing to shoulder as much of the burden as possible, but you can't do that if you're not treated well.

Advocate Tip #9 (page 38)
Get Dressed

Getting dressed up for doctors' appointments can help you and your patient feel more upbeat and positive, and possibly result in better treatment.

Advocate Tip #10 (page 43)
Make Use of the Internet

In your search for information, log on to Google and type in your illness, a treatment, or a procedure. Also try medlineplus.gov, a site run by the National Institutes of Health. If you're too intimidated, ask a computer-savvy friend or family member to help.

Advocate Tip #11 (page 45)
Address the Question of Faith

Be open to whatever your patient and you are feeling when it comes to faith, and know that in times of serious illness, ideas about faith may shift and change.

Advocate Tip #12 (page 48)
Find Physicians with a Team Approach

When you're gathering information from various physicians, ask them if they use a team approach. A true team approach means that the same group of people—surgeons, anesthesiologists, nurses— consistently work together in providing treatment and handling procedures for patients.

Advocate Tip #13 (page 50)
Put the Battle Plan into Action

Follow up on researching your patient's disease, getting second opinions from a variety of doctors, doing what you can to support your patient's immune system at home, and contacting the people in your communication network.

Advocate Tip #14 (page 51)
Issue a Call to General Quarters

Put out the news of your patient's diagnosis to everyone you know— and beyond. Someone you least expect may come up with a lead that will help tremendously.

Advocate Tip #15 (page 55)
Get Copies of Records

Ask for a release form and have your patient sign it, stating that you are authorized to have access to all records. *Don't* buy into the false idea that these records belong to the hospital or the medical provider. With MRIs and CT scans, you want the scans themselves, not just a written report.

Advocate Tip #16 (page 57)
Bum a Ride

For a list of several organizations that provide patients with flights in small jets for no cost, see page 212. You can also find a resource there for free lodging options when you arrive.

Get Your Patient Together with Friends

Do everything in your power to gather up those people you know will do your patient good. Who would your patient enjoy seeing and for what activities? If he or she can't get out, would your patient enjoy being in contact with them via the Internet?

Get a Second—or Even Third—Opinion

Don't get a second opinion from within the same medical group, or even at the same hospital. If possible at all, try to get an opinion from physicians in another city, who may tend to think differently.

Go for It When the Treatment Sounds Right

When your patient comes to believe in a treatment or specific doctor or facility, it's time to overcome your own concerns and back him up 100 percent.

Set Short-Term Goals and Rewards

Have something dangling out in front of your patient that can provide a positive focus during his or her dark moments. Whether it's a vacation or the birth of a grandchild or attending an important reunion, giving your patient something specific to look forward to is so important.

Make Use of a University-Affiliated Medical Center

These institutions usually have teaching and research facilities that may give you your best shot at cutting-edge technology.

Find Your Own Voice as an Advocate

Whether you're shy or outgoing, talkative or taciturn, be yourself. But above all, be an advocate.

Know Your Patient's Wishes

Have this difficult conversation with your patient early on. What extraordinary measures, if any, does he want taken to prolong life? Does she want to be on a respirator? When, if ever, does he want the "plug pulled"? Make sure your patient has a power of attorney in place for health care decisions.

Push the Envelope

Take a look at all the newer options. That means exploring clinical trials. See page 211 for resources on clinical trials.

Don't Try to Control Everything

Remind yourself over and over again that you can do your very best, try your hardest, and still not be able to guarantee a good outcome. Be gentle with yourself. No matter how hard you try, you can't control everything.

Advocate Tip #26 (page 86)
Make Doctors Speak in Language You Understand

Ask, "Doctor, could you please explain that to me slowly and in English so that I can understand what you are saying?" You need to understand what's happening to your patient in no uncertain terms.

Advocate Tip #27 (page 93)
Be Open to Complementary Alternative Medicine (CAM)

Look into nutrition, chiropractic, acupuncture, and other alternative treatments that will complement your doctors' treatment plans. See page 212 for resources on CAM for cancer patients. What complementary alternative treatments are appropriate for your patient?

Advocate Tip #28 (page 96)
Create a Stress-Free Environment

Make a list of all the things, from handling calls to safeguarding sleep, that you can do to create a relaxing environment for your patient. Then implement them.

Advocate Tip #29 (page 97)
Help Your Patient Get His or Her Affairs in Order

Make sure that your patient has legal and/or estate planning documents in order. Take the time to help your patient gather together all the documents an attorney will need to look at—documents like home deeds, insurance papers, how an IRA is held. Have your patient talk to the human resources person at his or her place of work. Start with a to-do list.

Advocate Tip #30 (page 98)
Pay Attention to the Medical Bills

Not all bills need to be paid immediately. Being organized in this area will relieve tremendous pressure. If it's too overwhelming, contact a for-profit company that will review your records for medical billing errors and also work to correct insurance billing mistakes. See page 213 for resources. For help with disputes about insurance coverage, contact your state insurance department.

Advocate Tip #31 (page 101)
Make Memories and Share Stories

Encourage your patient to use whatever media they're attracted to, whether video, audio, scrapbooks, or journals, to record and share the gift of their wisdom and the highlights of their lives with those they may leave behind.

Advocate Tip #32 (page 105)

Ask Questions—Constantly

Doctors and hospitals make mistakes, and it's the advocate's job to ask questions diligently at all times (see pages 106–7 for a complete list). And don't forget to write down the answers.

Advocate Tip #33 (page 110)

Don't Schedule Surgery During the Holidays

If it's not an absolute emergency, have surgery scheduled before or after holidays. This is the time when many medical personnel take their vacations. Make sure that you ask for the A-team.

Advocate Tip #34 (page 115)

Be There

Whenever your patient is in the hospital, you as the advocate need to be there right by his or her side. It is vital to maintain as much of a presence as you can.

Advocate Tip #35 (page 117)

How to Live Through a Hospital Experience

See pages 117–19 for a complete list of tips to make your patient's stay more comfortable. Add your own ideas, too.

Advocate Tip #36 (page 122)

Don't Take No as Their Final Answer

If you believe your patient needs something that's being denied him or her, push for what is needed. No matter what kind of resistance you meet, you always have legal recourse, and reminding hospitals and doctors' offices of this can be an effective last resort.

Advocate Tip #37 (page 123)

Bring the Comforts of Home

When your patient is in the hospital, bring photos of the family, cards made by grandkids, comfy pajamas, a bathrobe, and slippers. Bring a small DVD player, movies, music, and books. If appropriate, bring good food that meets your patient's dietary needs.

Advocate Tip #38 (page 128)

Put a Face on Your Disease

Whether you see Pac-Men eating cancer cells or nerve endings blooming like flowers, put a face on the condition so you can visualize exactly what the body needs to do to get better. How do you and your patient visualize the condition? How do you visualize its cure?

Advocate Tip #39 (page 137)

Get a Dog

I think that if you and/or your patient are in a position to have a dog or other pet, the journey through illness can only be made easier by its presence. If you can't own a pet, try to have regular contact with someone else's.

Advocate Tip #40 (page 139)
Treat Doctors, Nurses, and Medical Staff Well

To ensure the best treatment for your patient, try to make the medical professionals see you as individuals first. Ask them about their lives, be helpful, and "make friends" whenever possible.

Advocate Tip #41 (page 145)
Get Others to Help

Whom do you know who can offer a kind word or some specific help? Give those people a call.

Advocate Tip #42 (page 148)
Take Care of Yourself

Someone really needs to be looking out for the advocate, and while others can help, the person who can do that best is you, yourself. Take time off, get some exercise, eat well, and give yourself little treats. By taking care of yourself, you can take better care of your patient. How can you take care of yourself?

Advocate Tip #43 (page 152)
Get Private or Semi-Private Therapy

If you have the financial capability, this is a time when you need to open your wallet and pay for this extra expense on your own. Or borrow if you have to. High-quality recuperative therapy will affect your loved one every day for the rest of his or her life, and your life as well. Find out what kind of therapy your patient needs, who's the best provider, and brainstorm on how you'll pay for it.

Advocate Tip #44 (page 155)
Gather Inspirational Stories

Bring your patient inspirational stories, whether in book or movie form, of other people who used every ounce of their being to fortify themselves to keep putting one foot in front of the other until they got where they needed to be. What stories do you know that fit this description? See pages 216–18 for Brian's favorites.

Advocate Tip #45 (page 158)
Access Community Services

Every hospital or rehabilitation facility has a social worker who can help you get started finding resources in your community that will support your patient's recovery. Make a list of them.

Advocate Tip #46 (page 160)
Help Maintain Your Patient's Dignity

Ensure that the independence and pride of your patient are preserved as much as possible. From reading aloud in a casual way for someone who can't, to offering a subtle "hand-up" to a person whose mobility is compromised, note the little things you can do to help your loved one maintain dignity—and then do them.

Advocate Tip #47 (page 161)
Reach Out to Other Advocates

Whom do you know who has been through what you're going through now? You will find these folks can offer an empathetic shoulder to lean on when you need it most.

Advocate Tip #48 (page 165)
Celebrate the Milestones

It makes far more sense to spend money on a party than a funeral. Whether it's ending a round of chemotherapy or radiation, or reaching any other medical milestone, recognizing the value of these achievements gives your patient a huge psychological boost. What are your patient's milestones? How do you want to celebrate them?

Advocate Tip #49 (page 170)
Remember, This Is Not a Dress Rehearsal

Don't be overprotective. Let your loved one live life to the fullest, rather than languishing in the wings, waiting for the curtain to fall. What are those things you can do together to live to the fullest?

Advocate Tip #50 (page 172)
Always Think in Terms of "We"

As an advocate, think of yourself as part of a team. As far as it is humanly possible, see your patient's fight as your fight: no one has a more vested interest in winning the war than you. Jot down a few slogans to help you win the campaign against your opponent, the disease.

Patient's Medical History

We've found that it's vitally important to keep an updated copy of the patient's medical history on hand. This is the best way to ensure that doctors get the complete, accurate information they need to provide optimal care. It will also give you the peace of mind that comes from knowing you haven't forgotten any significant details, especially considering the stress you're under.

The following is an example of a basic medical history. Don't, however, regard these categories as definitive. Be sure to include any information you think might help a doctor better understand your patient's medical history.

Personal Data

Name: _____

Address: _____

_____

Phone numbers: _____

_____

Social Security number: _____

Name and phone numbers of person to contact in case of emergency: _____

_____

Primary care doctor and phone number: _____

_____

Insurance Information

Company, agent, phone numbers, policy numbers: _____

_____

_____

Doctors Seen Since Diagnosis

Name, specialty, phone number: _____

_____

_____

Name, specialty, phone number: _____

_____

_____

Name, specialty, phone number: _____

_____

_____

Name, specialty, phone number: _____

_____

_____

Significant Medical History

Including pregnancies, short- and long-term illnesses, heart conditions, high or low blood pressure, diabetes, high cholesterol, cancer, chronic illness, HIV/AIDS, or other conditions:_____

_____

_____

_____

_____

_____

_____

_____

_____

_____

Personal Habits

How much you smoke, drink, exercise: _____

_____

_____

Current Medications

Pharmacy and phone number: _____

Names of medications, who prescribed, doses, when began, when taken, side effects: _____

_____

_____

_____

_____

_____

Over-the-Counter Products

Including vitamins, supplements, herbs: _____

_____

_____

_____

_____

_____

Allergies

To medicines, foods, natural and man-made substances, insects, anything else that causes an unusual reaction, and how your body responds: _____

_____

_____

_____

_____

Hospitalizations

Including in-patient stays, out-patient procedures, ER visits:_____

_____

_____

_____

_____

_____

_____

Surgeries

Major and minor, including dates, hospitals, surgeons, problems with anesthesia, or any other complications: _____

_____

_____

_____

_____

_____

Recent Blood Tests

Get a copy of recent blood work, such as glucose, fasting cholesterol, white blood cell count, cancer values, kidney function, etc.: _____

_____

_____

_____

_____

_____

Special Tests and Procedures

X-rays, EKG, stress test, echocardiogram, colonoscopy, etc.: _____

_____

_____

_____

_____

_____

Family History

Significant diseases of grandparents, parents, siblings, children, including cause of death if applicable: _____

_____

_____

_____

_____

_____

Injuries, Accidents, Disabilities

And how they were treated: _____

_____

_____

_____

_____

_____

_____

Current Problems

Including symptoms: _____

_____

_____

_____

_____

_____

_____

_____

_____

_____

Any Other Information You Think Is Pertinent

Psychological problems, sleep disturbances, phobias, etc.: _____

_____

_____

_____

Living Through the Hospital Experience

Being in a hospital is a difficult situation for anyone. It can be especially daunting if your treatment requires numerous stays in different hospitals, and perhaps different cities. From our years of experience, we've learned some things that helped ease our way and, we think, even helped Brian get better care.

- First rule: get out of there as soon as possible!
- Don't schedule surgery during the holidays.
- In teaching hospitals, try to avoid the summer months, when the new interns have just made their way into hospital life. We know that they are there to learn, but our philosophy is to let them practice on someone else!
- Don't take no as a final answer when your patient needs assistance.
- Find out when your best chance to see the doctor is. When are morning rounds?
- Find out when the physical therapist, occupational therapist, or nutritionist will be there and make sure that you're there as well.
- Make friends with *everyone* who works in the hospital! Start by learning the names of the nurses and aides.
- Make certain that everyone who enters your patient's room washes his or her hands, staff included.
- Be there 24/7, or as much as you can.
- Bring comforts from home such as clothes, food, and photos.
- Find out where the nurses' station "kitchen" is, and offer to get water, ice, Jell-O, etc., for your patient.
- Find out where the linen closet is and get the extra bed pads, blankets, or pillows that your patient needs.
- Help with bathroom chores.
- Be extra vigilant when shifts change.

Gerri's Initial Battle Plan

Exhausted as I was that first night after Brian's diagnosis, I couldn't go to sleep. I knew we were going to war against cancer and we had to do everything in our power to win. So I got out a yellow legal pad and wrote out a plan of attack. Your battle plan will depend on the situation your patient is in, but these were my basics. If you find yourself in this situation, take the time to organize yourself. Perhaps you'll want spiritual support, maybe you'll need to reorganize your finances, but whatever it is *you* need to attack, write it down.

Research

What is this disease or condition your patient is facing? What can you do to learn everything you can about it? Who can help answer these questions?

_____

_____

_____

_____

_____

_____

_____

_____

Physicians

Who are the best physicians that specialize in this area? Whom do you know who can help put you in touch with the right physicians?

_____

_____

_____

_____

_____
_____
_____
_____
_____

Nutrition and Other Supplemental Care

What can you do to support your patient's immune system? What does his or her particular condition require? Who can help you answer these questions?

_____
_____
_____
_____
_____
_____
_____
_____
_____

Communication Network

List *all* the people who might want to or be able to help. In what ways might you rely on them? Setting up a telephone tree is vital, or you'll be worn out in no time from talking to everyone. E-mail lists are also a great way to keep people in the loop.

_____
_____
_____
_____
_____
_____
_____
_____
_____

Gerri's Personal Advocate's Notebook

The Advocate's Notebook I carried in my purse was my bible. It is a little 5- by 8-inch spiral notebook with pictures of sunflowers on the front, the kind you can find at any bookshop, pharmacy, or local discount store. But it contains an amazing amount of information and provides a running commentary on what has been going on with Brian. Your notebook will be different; it should be different—your patient is not Brian, and our situation is not yours.

Important Phone Numbers

The inside front and back covers of my book contain the names, addresses, and phone numbers of the doctors we saw. I also wrote down the names of the nurses and receptionists (it helped when I could ask for them by name). Because we went to so many places, this information spilled over to the pages at the back of the book.

Record of Appointments, Treatments, Medications

The pages beginning at the front contain dates and times of appointments with doctors, and what they said. There are notations such as "a vaccine might be a very reasonable approach," "melanoma gets good results from Gamma Knife radiation," and "recommends whole brain radiation." What was recommended and what they did to Brian ("needle biopsy of the tumor under his arm"), and the results ("he can't sleep, agitated, itching, scratching his head, his skin. Hiccups starting. Won't stop . . ."). I wrote down every medication he took and his reaction to it. I even wrote down his blood pressure after each procedure.

Practical Travel Information

Toward the back of the book, leaving room at the end for those important doctors' names, addresses, and phone numbers, I wrote down practical information that helped us as we traveled to various places for treatment. Phone numbers of cab companies in Dallas, San Francisco, etc. Hotel information. Places to eat. Written directions to doctors' offices in various cities. Phone numbers for airlines. 203

My notebook is nothing professional, but every advocate I know, and every patient we have befriended in the past ten years, has adopted something very similar to this. The importance is not what the notebook looks like—it simply needs to contain information to help make life easier for the advocate, and provide a running commentary of what is going on with the patient. Above all, it needs to be easy to carry so that it's accessible at all times.

The Lance Armstrong Foundation has created a thorough, very well thought out journal called the Survivorship Notebook, which can be obtained free of charge (you pay only shipping and handling) through their website, www.livestrong.org. It features printed versions of the information, worksheets, and stories found on their website.

Insights from Others

During our long and difficult battle, we were blessed by the friendships and understanding of people who supported and encouraged us, who were there with us and thus were part of our struggle. Now several of them offer their insights into particular moments and provide their perspectives as to why we were able to accomplish what we did.

How Brian Wrote the Ending First

Sherry Bahrambeygui, Law Partner

Doing anything for Brian Monaghan was not for the faint of heart. For Brian it was never just a case, it was a cause; never just a client, but a member of his family; never just litigation, but war. His fierce beliefs became yours, and his crusade on behalf of clients became your mission in life. Working for Brian was an all-consuming professional experience, one that—if it didn't kill you—made you into a passionate lawyer who recognized what an honor and awesome responsibility it is to help people who have been wronged.

In the process I also found one of the best friends of my life—a demanding man full of boundless generosity, who at the same time that he was fighting for his own survival, still had enough left to 204 support and inspire those around him.

I began to learn about Brian before I even met him. He was resented by those he had opposed, and revered by the rest. He powered a small firm known for beating the unbeatable giants, time and time again. When I was still a relatively new lawyer, I was approached about working with him. I didn't know what to expect at my job interview—frankly, the thought was a bit intimidating. But behind a rather large desk sat a casually clothed teddy bear. I recall leaving the four-hour interview exhausted, baffled, and intrigued. I would later learn that this was the exact process he would put each of his potential clients through in order to squeeze out all the facts and information he could, before making the commitment to represent someone. This was part of how he got to truly know his clients.

One of the first lessons Brian taught me was that early in a case, I should write the ending first. "How would you argue this in closing to a jury?" he would ask. I remember feeling frustrated at times, that it was too soon for me to know how everything should turn out. Brian's lesson was simple: if you do not have a clear image of where you are headed, you will not know how to get there. Whether you call it vision, drive, or faith, Brian had an uncanny ability to see how things should turn out with amazing clarity and conviction. He would often write the ending first, and as he undertook the process, he would uncover every piece of information and bit of evidence that advanced the goal. It was this clarity and focus that helped Brian overcome inevitable setbacks in trial as well as in his fight against cancer.

What Brian taught me was that much of where you end up is based on your genuine faith in the outcome, and that by writing the ending first, you can influence your own destiny.

How Gerri Used Courage and Tenacity

Daniel Einhorn, M.D., Medical Director
of the Scripps Whittier Institute for Diabetes

When I called to get the results of Brian's MRI, the neurologist on the phone was matter-of-fact.

"Yes, we found something in the brain. Looks like cancer."

Silence.

Then I made frantic phone calls to question the evidence, to somehow find another explanation—but no, it was undeniable—even though I'd known something was very wrong from the outset. I think Gerri did, too. Brian wasn't thinking about it yet.

Little did he know, Gerri was about to save his life.

I knew they were waiting for the test results, and I struggled with how to break the news. I telephoned to ask Gerri and Brian to meet me at the office, a request that in itself began to prepare them.

At the office I tried to soften the news with language like "This is preliminary," and "There are many possibilities," but Gerri would have none of it. She was like a laser beam. In the moment of that first mention of "something on the x-ray," Gerri understood.

There is no more chilling news than to be told you have a metastatic melanoma to the brain, and courage was one blessing I wished for them. I was about to be given a lesson in another most precious blessing—tenacity.

Gerri became the world's authority on who was doing what for metastatic melanoma. At one point, she knew more than anyone about what was happening in this labyrinthine and often contradictory field where there is no single authority, no single answer. And nothing was impossible, no treatment inaccessible, if it could save her Brian.

In this she taught me another critical blessing—ferocity. If raw power has the capacity to heal, Gerri healed Brian.

The healing continues. And the healing has extended to friends and family who are enriched and forever grateful to have shared this miracle.

How Mom and Brian Trusted Their Instincts

Todd Wortmann, Gerri's Son

I have to admit that I was a little spooked about going on the trip to San Francisco for another "second opinion." We were in constant communication with Mom, getting all the updates, good and bad, about the various places they were going to seek medical advice. Although she always tried to sound upbeat and positive, I could hear the strain in her voice leading up to this trip. I had talked to

everyone I knew in the medical field, and they all told me the same thing: Brian's diagnosis was about as bad as it could get. Jennifer and I talked about the fact that it all seemed so unfair. Brian and Mom had really just started a life together and now it seemed like there wouldn't be much of a future for them. But they were both clear that they weren't giving in. They had two things going for them. Brian's attitude was one of complete optimism, and I knew that in this fight he had a secret weapon in his corner—my mom. Even with that, there was no doubt it was getting scary; the days were flying by much too quickly. I was hoping, almost counting on the docs at UCSF to be the ones who could help them.

After getting lost on our way from the airport and hitting the streets of San Francisco in our slapstick version of a chase scene from a Dirty Harry movie, we arrived at one beaten down, ugly-looking hospital. The building itself sure didn't give anyone a sense of confidence. But within ten minutes of the first meeting of that long day, I had a feeling that Brian and Mom had found the place that held the answers. Both of them tend to get quiet when things aren't going right, but they weren't quiet now. Mom began peppering the doctor with questions and they kept turning to each other and giving each other little nods. I swear that I could hear the sound of hope beginning to come through in their voices. At one point later in the day, Brian and I were alone in a room and he asked me what I thought. "It seems like you connected with these docs right off the bat in a way that you didn't at the other places." We went through some quick pros and cons and I told him that I thought this was the place to get it done. Brian nodded and said he had the same feeling. Watching Brian and Mom react in such a positive way to the people they were dealing with, instead of focusing on the bleakness of the surroundings, was a powerful lesson for me to watch in action. Trust your instincts.

Don't Give Up Too Soon

Dr. Maurizio Zanetti, M.D., University of California, San Diego

There was no magic message I could deliver to Brian and Gerri when we met not long after his diagnosis. There was no idea of what to do, either. So going back to what I had learned in medical school, I used a small blackboard to construct a grid that listed the current therapeutic options available in the field I knew best, immunotherapy. In doing so, I realized how far behind we were in translating cutting-edge science into opportunities for patients.

When Brian and Gerri left, it was obvious to me that the most important thing was to infuse them with an element of hope that something was going to be done. The assurance that there may exist a way out builds new energy in a patient, and a sense of confidence that is so important for enduring the dark times patiently, one at a time, going forward and not giving in.

The task of finding a viable option was difficult, but after a series of phone calls, I contacted the group at Baylor University Medical Center in Dallas, Texas, which was just about ready to begin a clinical study on dendritic-cells/peptide vaccination in melanoma. Baylor had not yet begun enrolling anyone in the program and the eligibility criteria seemed to be all right for Brian. More than that, it looked as if an element of luck was with him. By absolute chance, the clinician in charge of the trial, Dr. Joe Fay, was vacationing in San Diego; when I contacted him, he was willing to take the time to meet with us and discuss Brian's chances to be enrolled. The prospect of being part of the trial became instantly more realistic.

Brian's story shares many components with the stories of other cancer patients. There are thousands of Brians in the world who find themselves at the same crossroad every day. That moment is painful, filled with confusion, uncertainty, impotence, and despair. Brian saw that the course of things could be reversed and that ultimately life could return to a level of normality when two factors started to play in unison: the prospect of the new treatment, and a strong will to fight and prevail. Brian's story is the story of hope and courage—of not closing the door too soon.

How to Support a Positive Attitude
Kathi Vaughn, Brian's Daughter

My parents divorced when I was eleven, and after that my brother and I lived with our father. Life was often filled with spontaneity and laughter. Dad was constantly making us laugh with his imaginative bedtime fairy tales, and embarrassing us with his loud singing in public. I'll always be amazed by his ability to juggle being an involved single parent and a successful attorney. At times it must have been a struggle for him, but we never experienced that side: he always made things fun. I knew that my father worked very hard as an attorney, and I knew that when he went off to court he always remained confident, even in the face of the toughest situations. Sometimes his absolute confidence may have been contrived for our benefit, but it worked for our family and we always felt that things would be okay.

It was the same when he told me he had cancer. Our family wasn't a stranger to cancer—we had seen several relatives struggle and lose their battle with it. But I believed if anyone could defeat this devastating disease, my father could. He and I had always talked about everything, and that didn't change when he was diagnosed. My dad never once spoke of dying. His attitude was, "I'm going to beat this!" And I had no reason to doubt him.

Of course I knew there would be difficult times ahead. Now the tables were turned, and it was up to me to be the one with absolute confidence. Cancer is stressful, and during the most difficult times it is important to believe in a person's strength and ability to fight. It is also crucial to create a peaceful environment. As loved ones struggle to cope, anxiety levels rise, creating tension among family members. This is when to let the little things go and keep the patient a priority. This is also the time to break the rules. I smuggled my son into the hospital for a visit, and it ended up being one of my dad's most memorable moments.

My hope for people battling cancer (or any other disease) is that they have an advocate as wonderful as Gerri, a positive attitude and a will as strong as my father's, and the love and support of family and friends.

A Dream Yet to Be Realized

Dr. Jacques Banchereau, Ph.D., Director of the
Baylor Institute for Immunology Research

I have to admit that when we injected Brian with the dendritic-cell vaccine, it almost made me cry. Everybody was very, very touched. Brian represented a strong incentive for us to continue our ceaseless labors, because these moments of reward are precious few. We have since injected more than eighty patients and we see progress. As scientists, however, we won't believe we have achieved complete success until the vaccine is available on a wide scale to everybody. It is a goal we hope to reach within the next three years. If that happens, it will be the culmination of a twenty-year effort.

Why Did Brian Make It?

Dr. Mike McDermott, Director of Gamma Knife Radiosurgery,
Vice Chairman of the Department of Neurological Surgery,
UCSF Medical Center

One of the things I would say about Brian and Gerri Monaghan is that they have approached the problem of fighting cancer with an upbeat and positive attitude. At the same time they accepted that there are certain trials and tribulations associated with this battle—the necessary penance for the surgical interventions that by most would be regarded as aggressive. Nonetheless, the treatments to date have proven to be effective, and Brian is one of the lucky few who have survived a lengthy time after their original diagnosis of multiple brain metastases.

The oncology literature notes that patients who are involved in support groups and those who enter clinical trials generally do better than patients who do not. Although the medical therapy offered through these programs no doubt had an influence on the outcome, there are other, less tangible factors that must be playing a role. The nurturing support of a close-knit family obviously reduces stress, and this almost certainly has an effect on the outcome. The ability to live each day looking forward with a positive attitude, I think, has also helped Brian. Many of us take things for granted and it's only, unfortunately, after a serious illness that we realize how precious each day is. Physicians need to remember, too, that all the technology we have may not always be successful in eradicating tumors.

I believe that the patient plays a significant role in influencing the biology of the body's reaction, surveillance, and response to tumors. Brian always jokes that it's the Bushmills that has kept his melanoma away, but I think it's his outgoing, fun-loving spirit that's the key.

210

Brian and Gerri's Idiosyncratic Catchall of Helpful Resources and Information

Here is a very loosely organized compendium of practical information, websites, inspirations, and other resources we hope will empower you in the struggle ahead. Again, many of our resources had to do with cancer. You'll need to adapt for your particular situation.

Brian and Gerri's Website

Many of the cancer resources referred to below can be explored via links from our website, www.ReadthePoweroffTwo.com.

Treatment Plans and Other Resources for Cancer Patients

The American Cancer Society has a helpful website, www .cancer.org, as well as people staffing their phone lines twenty-four hours a day (800-ACS-2345) who are willing to give advice on where to start your search.

A Citizens' Cancer Lobby

To support political efforts to fund cancer research and to support and organize events in your community, contact:
- **The Lance Armstrong Foundation:** www.livestrong.org
- **American Cancer Society Cancer Action Network:** www.acscan.org

Finding Out About Clinical Trials

There are several government-sponsored websites that have information on clinical trials, but a good place to start is this registry of federally and privately funded clinical trials in the U.S. and abroad:
- **ClinicalTrials.gov:** www.clinicaltrials.gov. This website contains information on clinical trials relating to virtually every type of disease or condition.

Several organizations offer information about clinical trials for cancer patients in particular, among them:

- **Coalition of Cancer Cooperative Groups:** 877-520-4457; www.cancertrialshelp.org
- **National Comprehensive Cancer Network:** 888-909-6226; www.nccn.org
- **American Cancer Society:** 800-ACS-2345; www.cancer.org

Complementary Alternative Medicine for Cancer Patients

If you go to the website www.cancer.org, you can check on the viability of alternative treatments for various types and stages of cancer.

Air Transportation Options

Several charitable organizations will allow you to bum a ride to medical centers around the country. An extensive list of websites relating to free flights for patients in need in different parts of the country can be found at www.medscape.com. Also contact:

- **Air Charity Network:** 877-621-7177; www.airlifeline.org
- **Angel Flight Mid-Atlantic:** 800-296-3797; www.angelflight midatlantic.org
- **Corporate Angel Network:** 866-328-1313; www.corpangel network.org
- **National Patient Travel Center:** 800-296-1217; www.patient travel.org

Since we intended to continue traveling for pleasure as much as possible, we joined Medjet Assistance, a company that provides medical transportation and assistance throughout the world during a medical crisis. They will immediately send assistance to distant locations, and then transport the patient to the appropriate medical facility. For instance, if we were in some godforsaken place and a medical crisis occurred, they would send a private plane with a doctor or nurse to transport Brian to our hospital in San Diego. The annual cost is about $400 for a family. Like most insurance, the hope is that you will never need to use it, and thus far, we haven't had to, but our awareness of its existence has given us (especially Gerri) a great sense of comfort. More specifics are available at www.medjetassistance.com or 800-5-ASSIST.

Lodging Options

The National Association of Hospital Hospitality Houses provides information regarding lodging assistance for patients and others traveling for medical emergencies. Their website is www.nahhh.org.

Canine Companions

Some organizations with information regarding assistance dogs:
- **Canine Companions for Independence:** www.caninecompanions.org
- **Assistance Dogs International:** www.assistance-dogs-intl.org
- **Guiding Eyes for the Blind:** www.guidingeyes.org

Help in Organizing and Paying Medical Bills

For support in making sure you don't pay any more than you have to, check out Medical Billing Advocates of America: 540-387-5870; www.billadvocates.com. Although it deals specifically with Medicare information, the California Health Advocates website, www.cahealthadvocates.org, has a section on organizing and dealing with medical bills that is very helpful in regard to *any* medical bills.

Help in Fighting Insurance Companies

Contact your state insurance department or commissioner to see if they can provide assistance if your patient is denied medical coverage or if payments have been capped. The Patient Advocate Foundation is a nonprofit group with volunteer attorneys and other professionals who can help mediate insurance disputes. Contact them at www.patientadvocate.org.

Resources for Long-Term Care

If you need support for the arduous task of caring for your loved one at home, check out these organizations:
- **Lotsa Helping Hands:** www.lotsahelpinghands.com
- **National Alliance for Caregiving:** www.caregiving.org
- **National Family Caregivers Association:** 800-896-3650; www.thefamilycaregiver.org
- **The Wellness Community:** www.thewellnesscommunity.org

213

- **Share the Care:** 646-467-8097; www.sharethecare.org
- **Well Spouse Association:** 800-838-0879; www.wellspouse.org
- **The Wellness Community:** 888-739-WELL; www.thewellness community.org

Gamma Knife Surgery

You can find a precise, detailed explanation of the Gamma Knife procedure at the University of California San Francisco website (www.ucsfhealth.org) by typing "gamma knife" in the search box. The medically correct term for the procedure is "stereotactic radiosurgery." It's really not surgery at all, but rather a noninvasive technique for treating tumors that was developed by a Swedish neurosurgeon and first used in Sweden in 1951. Unfortunately, it took more than thirty-five years before this procedure gained acceptance in this country.

Technology has taken huge steps in the last ten years, and the medical field is no different. American Radiosurgery now manufactures a new instrument, the Rotating Gamma System. With it, the patient no longer has to be put into one of the huge helmets, and since the beams of radiation can be controlled internally, the procedures can be performed much faster. The first of these systems was installed in Chicago in 2003, and the latest one in San Diego in 2008. The neurosurgeons now utilizing this equipment believe that the newer technology and unique rotating design provide them with an increased ability to target brain disorders not previously recognized with other noninvasive treatment options. They believe that the Rotating Gamma System enables them to treat tumors that are deeper within the brain, and allows for increased protection of surrounding brain tissue. You can check this out at their website, www.americanradiosurgery.net.

Understanding Dendritic Cells

Dr. Jacques Banchereau, the director of the Baylor Institute for Immunology Research, described dendritic cells to us as the "generals of the immune-system army." His article on dendritic cells, "The Long Arm of the Immune System," published in the

November 2002 issue of *Scientific American,* can be found at the publication's website: www.sciamdigital.com. An excerpt reads:

> They lie buried—their long, tentacle-like arms outstretched—in all the tissues of our bodies that interact with the environment. In the lining of our nose and lungs, lest we inhale the influenza virus in a crowded subway car. In our gastrointestinal tract, to alert our immune system if we swallow a dose of salmonella bacteria. And most important, in our skin, where they lie in wait as stealthy sentinels should microbes breach the leathery fortress of our epidermis.

The Baylor Institute for Immunology Research is a component of the Baylor Research Institute in Dallas. For more information, you can visit www.baylorhealth.com, or call 800-4-BAYLOR.

For more information on dendritic cells, you can also visit our website: www.ReadthePowerofTwo.com.

Tools for Help with the Aphasia Battle

One of the first things we did after Brian was diagnosed with aphasia was to contact agencies that deal with the blind; we knew Brian would be having some of the same types of problems that a blind person would encounter. A great place to start is www .brailleinstitute.org.

Like many other universities around the country, one of our local universities, San Diego State, has a reading service that is available free of charge. They supply a special radio, and a schedule of programs that can be heard only via that special radio. For example, between 8:00 and 11:00 in the morning, a volunteer will read articles from the specified newspapers, and the person with aphasia can either just listen or follow along.

For those who love to read, aphasia can be a severe blow that audio books can help alleviate. Most libraries now have a section devoted to audio books. There are also websites from which you can download audio books to an iPod. While buying audio books can be expensive, you can reduce the cost by purchasing them used over the Internet. Brian is constantly hooked up to an audio book and consumes them at an incredible rate. We have acquired boxes of these audio books over the last few years, and we make a point of donating many of them to our local library or the Center for the Blind. In addition, Brian keeps a catalog of the books he has and is more than happy to pass them along to friends and family.

The best tool we have found for Brian has been a computer program, AspireREADER 4.0, which actually reads aloud from almost any medium. While neither Brian nor I have any understanding of how it works, this program can read newspapers, magazines, or even things you've written yourself. For instance, loaded onto our computer are *The New York Times, Sports Illustrated, Time, Newsweek,* our local newspaper, and many other sources. Each day Brian can turn on our computer, select his newspaper or magazine, and then choose whatever article he wants to listen to. The program can be read in the pace, tone, volume, and even gender of the reader he chooses. The system is remarkable, and it costs only about $229. The extremely reasonable price is a result of public, private, and governmental support for individuals with disabilities. You can learn more about this product by visiting www.cast.org (search for AspireREADER). In partnership with Aequus Technologies, AspireREADER 4.0 provides "special features and navigation controls for individuals with sensory and cognitive disabilities."

If your patient has suffered a stroke, a valuable starting point for help and information is The National Stroke Association at www.stroke.org or 800-STROKES.

Brian's Inspirational Book Club

Each of these stories relates to the concept of courage and survival in different forms, and each of them meant a lot to Brian. Most are true, but a few are fiction. We hope you'll look beyond the "inspirational section" of the library or bookstore to find stories that touch your soul.

The Endurance: Shackleton's Legendary Antarctic Expedition by Caroline Alexander. Facing starvation and death, Shackleton "wrote his ending first" in exercising leadership and exceptional personal courage in reaching his goal. Although it took twenty months, he eventually led his men to safety.

It's Not About the Bike and *Every Second Counts* by Lance Armstrong. After his diagnosis of testicular cancer, Armstrong was willing to push the envelope to find the best treatment available. He also learned the lesson of paying it forward, and has since made a contribution to the world that goes far beyond any achievement he made as a cyclist.

Seabiscuit: An American Legend by Laura Hillenbrand. The story of a horseracing underdog and the group of misfits who came together to overcome the odds. But of equal importance to me was "A Conversation with Laura Hillenbrand" in the back of the book. While the author's chronic fatigue syndrome has limited her contact with the outside world, her courage and determination to write this book allowed her to find a way to reach out to others.

Between a Rock and a Hard Place by Aron Ralston. A twenty-eight-year-old climber gets his right arm trapped between a boulder and a canyon wall. For me, the story encapsulates the innate desire to live, the willingness to do whatever it takes to move forward with life, even if it means leaving part of yourself behind.

Ghost Soldiers: The Epic Account of World War II's Greatest Rescue Mission by Hampton Sides. This story of courage and survival amid unbelievable brutality recounts the lives of American soldiers who survived the atrocities of the Bataan Death March only to face three years of torment in a Japanese prison camp.

Gates of Fire: An Epic Novel of the Battle of Thermopylae by Steven Pressfield. A historical novel about 300 Spartans who held 100,000 invading Persians at bay. There was no question that the Spartans were about to die, but the story of their courage in the face of death and the choice they made in how to live their remaining time is truly inspiring.

Life of Pi by Yann Martel. Through an incredible set of circumstances, sixteen-year-old Pi finds himself adrift on a small raft in the middle of the Pacific, with an enormous Bengal tiger for company. While other readers have focused on the religious allegorical connection, I found the theme of using one's intellect to survive to be really compelling.

Brian's Do-It-Yourself Fairy Tale Kit

Brian loved to make up fairy tales for his children almost every night when they were growing up, and he'd always hoped that they would carry on the tradition when they had children of their own. Now, faced with the reality that time might be running out, Brian decided that he needed to write down the mechanics of how he had created these stories. At a time when the ravages of cancer were really taking a toll, this exercise in creative writing seemed to give him relief from some of the demons he was facing, and perhaps was a way to transport himself to a happier world—if only for a short while. After all, fantasy is a wonderful outlet for all of us.

Brian's Do-It-Yourself Fairy Tale Kit is the guide he put together to help Kathi and Patrick create their own stories for their kids. We offer it to you as a vehicle to create your own fantasy world for those who may follow. Could there possibly be a better way to pass along some happy memories?

When making up a fairy tale, tailor the story to your audience. In my case, I always had two main characters, a girl named Pickles (amazingly enough the same age and with the same physical description as my daughter) and a boy named Rocky (amazingly enough the same age and with the same physical description as my son). Central to each story was the inclusion of a "friend." In my case, I often used a unicorn that took the characters off to distant times and places and along the way imparted some much needed wisdom and advice. A magical element helps. Pickles and Rocky were able to travel using either the Magic Tree of Time or the Magic Waterfall (which allowed them to breathe underwater for exactly five hours). No fairy tale is complete without a villain and my favorite was The Screaming Yellow Zinger.

What comes around goes around and while I was ill, Sue Young Vaage, a longtime friend who knew of my love of fairy tales, created two for me. On learning of my cancer problem, Sue wrote "The

Ronin," the story of a samurai warrior who metaphorically fought a battle against cancer by using a sword called the Gamma Knifu, which drew its strength and power from the strength and will, the focus, and the inner peace of the samurai himself. After a long fight, Ronin vanquished the enemy and then retired to "The Temple of the Dragon Slayer." Reading these two fables brought tears to my eyes and helped see me through some of the dark hours. I recommend fairy tale therapy for all!

A Few of Brian's Irish Jokes

To us, laughter is one of life's greatest blessings, and even in the darkest of times we always seemed to find our sense of humor. Of course, it doesn't hurt that Brian is an Irishman . . . So here goes: Brian's all-time favorite jokes. May you enjoy a good laugh!

Confessional Sins

In the town of Galway lived Mickey Finnigan who was known as quite a rapscallion.

One Saturday afternoon, he entered the church and stepped into the confessional. "Please bless me, Father, for I have sinned. It has been four months since my last confession. These are my sins. I am terribly upset that I have been engaged in sexual sins with a woman here in the parish. Because these were sins of a terrible sexual nature, I am embarrassed to tell you her name."

The priest leaned closer and said, "Ah, now. You can speak to me, my son. Was it Bridgett Rafferty?"

"No, father. All these sins that I engaged in occurred many, many times and were very terrible in their sexuality."

"Oh, my son, was it Mary Kelley?"

"Father, I am even more ashamed to tell you."

"Well, my son, could it be it was Megan O'Flynn?"

"Father, I am so embarrassed that I've got to come back another time. I can't talk about it anymore."

As he was leaving the church, Mickey was approached by a friend who said, "Mickey, what the hell are you doing here? I haven't seen you in a church for years."

Mickey replied, "I'm just getting some leads."

The Seven Iron

Steve Conway and his son were on a golfing trip to Ireland and were playing one of the great courses, Ballybunion. They came to a hole where they had to hit over the water. The son asked his caddy for a seven iron. In his wonderful Irish brogue, the caddy replied.

"Ah, now, I don't believe that a seven iron will make it. I think you're going to need a five iron."

"No, give me the seven."

"Are you sure now?"

"Yes, give me the seven."

Just as the golfer lined up to hit the ball, the caddy called out, "Wait just a minute!"

He came over, knelt down close to the ball, and in a great stage whisper said, "Take a deep breath now."

He Didn't Mention Your Name

In the west of Ireland lived Seamus O'Foggerty. One evening as he came home to his little cottage and stepped through the door, he saw in the bedroom the sight of naked flesh! He rushed inside and there, standing stark naked in front of a mirror, was his wife of thirty years, Megan.

Seamus roared:"What the hell are you doin'?"

"Seamus, what a surprise. I went to the doctor today and he said to me, 'Megan, for a woman your age you have a beautiful body.' I was just standin' here in front of the mirror admiring me beautiful body."

"Did he say anything about your big fat arse?" asked Seamus.

"No, Seamus,"replied Megan. "He didn't mention your name at all."

Share a Drink with Me

At a narrow and dangerous curve in the north of Ireland, two cars sideswiped each other and went into a ditch. A Catholic priest crawled out from his car and went over to the opposing driver, who also just managed to slide out from beneath his car. The Catholic priest noticed immediately that the other driver was a Protestant

minister.

"Ah, Reverend, are you all right?"

"Ay, that I am. And you?"

"A few bumps and bruises, but I'll be fine. Is your car well?"

"Well, like your own; there seems to be a lot of damage, but it will do."

The Catholic priest then said, "Since our lives seem to have been spared by God, I think we should celebrate. I happen to have a bit of Irish whiskey here."

The minister took a sip and the priest suggested he have a bit more, as it was a lucky day for them, under the circumstances.

After a few more drinks the minister passed the bottle back to the priest and asked, "Now, will you have some yourself."

"Aye, that I will, but first I'll wait until after the police arrive to investigate the accident."

What a Coincidence!

In a pub in County Cork stood the bartender Timmy Rafferty. As he cleaned the beer glasses he overheard two gentlemen sitting across from each other at the corner of the bar. It sounded much like this:

"My name is Timmy. What's yours?"

"Johnny's me name."

"Where you from?"

"County Mayo."

"County Mayo? What a coincidence. I'm from County Mayo meself."

"Oh, we are now? Where did you go to school?"

"I went to St. Joseph's."

"St. Joseph's in County Mayo? Amazing! So did I!"

"When did you graduate?"

"1972."

"1972? So did I! Who was your homeroom teacher?"

"Sister Mary Eloise."

"Well, Sister Mary Eloise was my homeroom teacher. Doesn't that just beat it all?"

At about this time the phone rang. The bartender answered and said, "Ah, yea, it's a slow night. Not much goin' on. I've just got the Murphy twins here, and they're at it again!"